Skull Base Surgery

*Edited by Hamid Borghei-Razavi,
Mauricio Mandel and Eric Suero Molina*

Published in London, United Kingdom

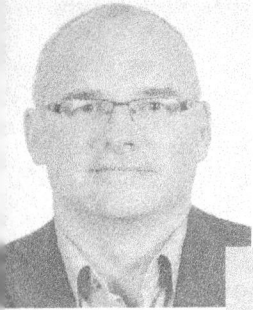
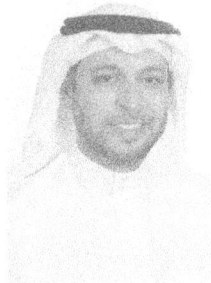
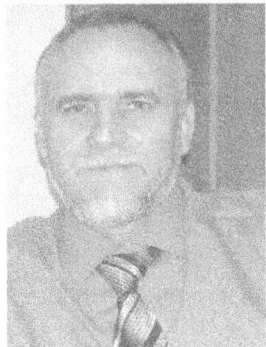
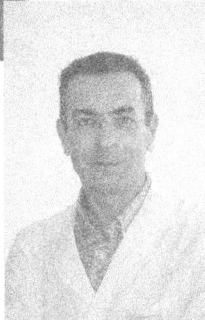
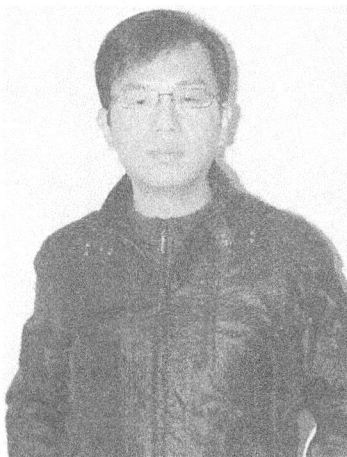
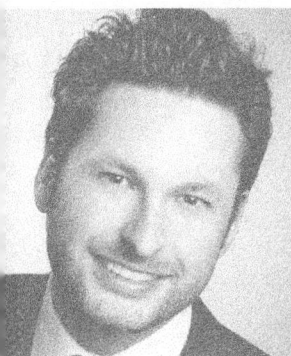
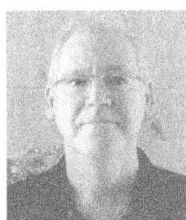

IntechOpen

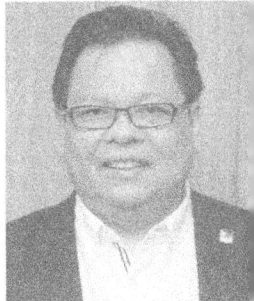
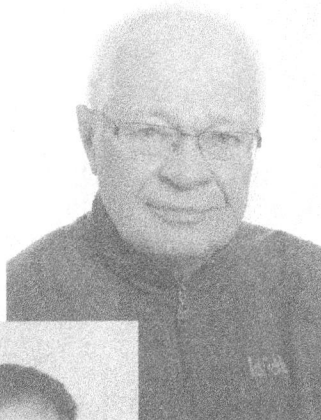
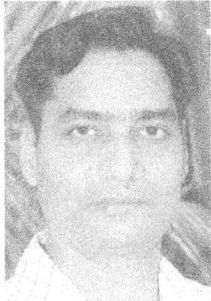
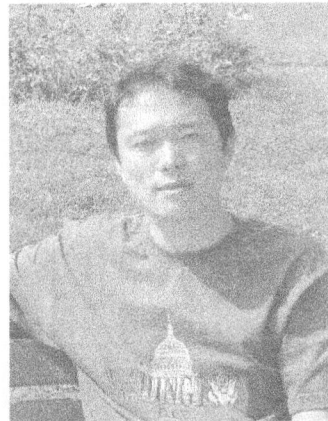
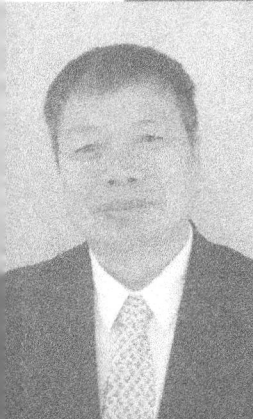
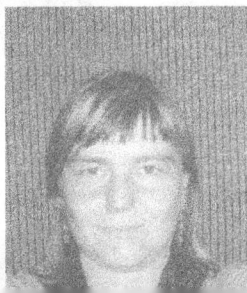

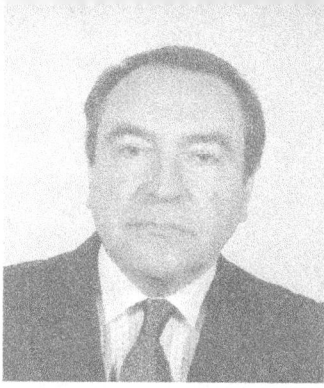

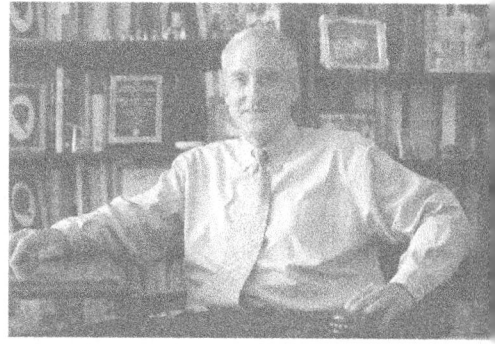

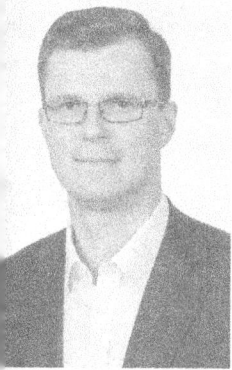

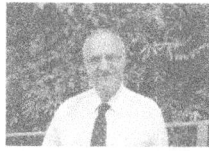

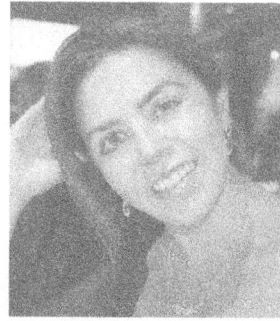

Supporting open minds since 2005

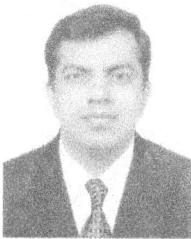

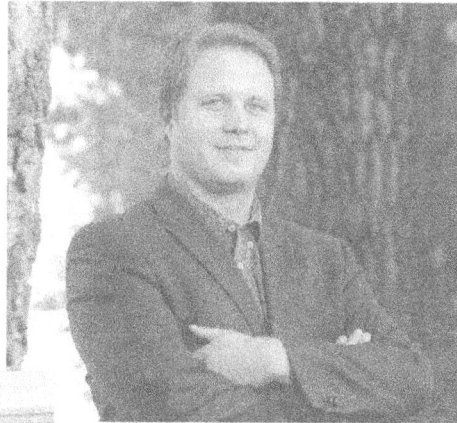

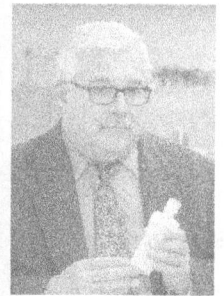

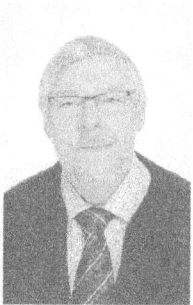

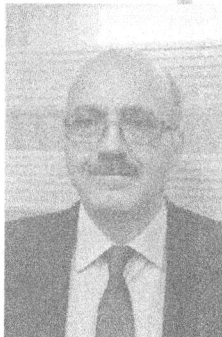

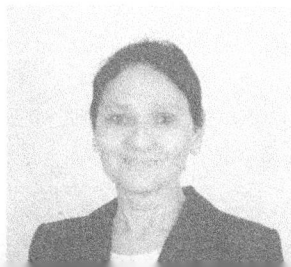

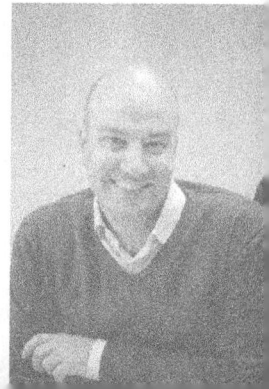

Skull Base Surgery
http://dx.doi.org/10.5772/intechopen.95175
Edited by Hamid Borghei-Razavi, Mauricio Mandel and Eric Suero Molina

Contributors
Kentaro Watanabe, Sébastien Froelich, Oleksandr Voznyak, Nazarii Hryniv, Arnar Astradsson, Amit Kumar Chowhan, Pavan Kumar G. Kale, Bilal Ibrahim, Hamid Borghei-Razavi, Mauricio Mandel, Assad Ali, Edison Najera, Michael Obrzut, Badih Adada, Uwe Spetzger, Julie Etingold, Andrej von Schilling, Guillaume Baucher, Pierre-Hugues Roche, Lucas Troude, Arsheed Hussain Hakeem, Hassaan Javaid, Novfa Iftikhar, Usaamah Javaid

Notice
Statements and opinions expressed in the chapters are these of the individual contributors and not necessarily those of the editors or publisher. No responsibility is accepted for the accuracy of information contained in the published chapters. The publisher assumes no responsibility for any damage or injury to persons or property arising out of the use of any materials, instructions, methods or ideas contained in the book.

First published in London, United Kingdom, 2022 by IntechOpen
IntechOpen is the global imprint of INTECHOPEN LIMITED, registered in England and Wales, registration number: 11086078, 5 Princes Gate Court, London, SW7 2QJ, United Kingdom
Printed in Croatia

British Library Cataloguing-in-Publication Data
A catalogue record for this book is available from the British Library

Additional hard and PDF copies can be obtained from orders@intechopen.com

Skull Base Surgery
Edited by Hamid Borghei-Razavi, Mauricio Mandel and Eric Suero Molina
p. cm.
Print ISBN 978-1-83962-632-6
Online ISBN 978-1-83962-633-3
eBook (PDF) ISBN 978-1-83962-634-0

We are IntechOpen,
the world's leading publisher of
Open Access books

Built by scientists, for scientists

6,100+
Open access books available

149,000+
International authors and editors

185M+
Downloads

Our authors are among the

156
Countries delivered to

Top 1%
most cited scientists

12.2%
Contributors from top 500 universities

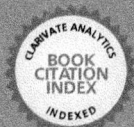

Interested in publishing with us?
Contact book.department@intechopen.com

Numbers displayed above are based on latest data collected.
For more information visit www.intechopen.com

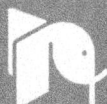

Meet the editors

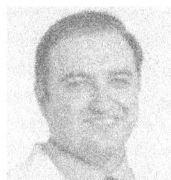

Hamid Borghei-Razavi, MD, is director of the Minimally Invasive Cranial and Pituitary Surgery Program at Cleveland Clinic Florida, research director of the Neuroscience Institute at Cleveland Clinic Florida Region, and Assistant Professor of Neurological Surgery at Cleveland Clinic Lerner College of Medicine. He specializes in brain tumor surgery, open and endoscopic skull base surgery, pituitary surgery, and trigeminal neuralgia. Dr. Borghei-Razavi received his medical degree from the Iran University of Medical Sciences (IUMS) and the University of Lübeck (Universität zu Lübeck), Germany. He completed his residency training at Clemenshospital, University of Münster, Germany. During his residency training, he was awarded a scholarship by the German Society of Neurosurgery (DGNC) to participate in a resident exchange program at the prestigious Keio University Skull Base Center, Tokyo, Japan. After finishing his training in Germany, he performed a yearlong research fellowship in skull base neuroanatomy at the University of Pittsburgh Medical Center (UPMC). He then completed two clinical fellowships in neurosurgical oncology and advanced open and endoscopic skull base surgery at Cleveland Clinic, Ohio, devoting his efforts to minimally invasive neurosurgical techniques.

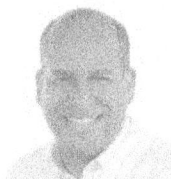

Dr. Suero-Molina is a staff neurosurgeon at the University Hospital Münster, Germany, and the head of minimally invasive endoscopic and endonasal skull base and orbital surgery. His residency and later his fellowship in neuro-oncology and complex skull base tumors occurred in the same department at the University Hospital of Münster. He is also on the clinical staff of neuro-oncology and spine surgery at the University of Münster.

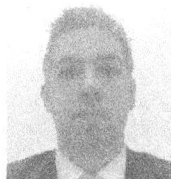

Dr. Mauricio Mandel obtained his medical degree at the University of Sao Paulo, Brazil, and did his neurosurgery residency at Hospital das Clínicas, University of Sao Paulo Medical School. Upon graduation, he received the "Edmundo Vasconcelos" prize as the best student in all surgical disciplines. Additionally, Dr. Mandel obtained a clinical Ph.D. in Minimally Invasive Neurosurgery at the University of Sao Paulo in 2018. He worked as an attending neurosurgeon at Hospital Israelita Albert Einstein, Sao Paulo, and Hospital das Clinicas of the University of Sao Paulo from 2010 to 2019. In 2019, Dr. Mandel moved to the United States and joined Stanford University, California, as a clinical instructor. He underwent further training in epilepsy surgery at Yale University, Connecticut. Currently, he is working in the Department of Neurosurgery, Cleveland Clinic Florida-Martin Health with a focus on minimally invasive neurosurgery (cranial and spine surgery).

Contents

Preface

Modern skull base surgery has developed into a multidisciplinary specialty with a specific collaboration between several diagnostic and therapeutic medical disciplines. It has undergone substantial evolution over the past 30 years. Although resection of skull base tumors was sporadically attempted in the early part of the 20th century, it was not until the 1960s that interest in the management of skull base tumors was piqued by the introduction and subsequent rapid expansion of indications of transnasal endoscopic techniques.

In parallel, extraordinary progress has been made in all the other disciplines (pathology, radiology, neurosurgery, radiation oncology, medical oncology) involved in the complex process of managing anterior skull base tumors, leading to substantial improvements in diagnosis and treatment. Due to complex anatomy and important functional structures, there are specific conditions for surgical procedures at the skull base. They require a maximum of precision, persistency, and well-grounded anatomical knowledge.

This book includes chapters written by experts worldwide. In view of the extreme variability of lesions involving the skull base, much emphasis has been placed on addressing the different nuances of treatment in relation to histology. The chapters focusing on surgery reflect the experience of the senior author and consequently provide divergent views on selection criteria for a specific surgical technique. The book contains a great deal of information on the topic of skull base tumors that is normally only available in journal articles.

Hamid Borghei-Razavi and Mauricio Mandel
Cleveland Clinic Florida,
Weston, Florida, USA

Eric Suero Molina
University Hospital Muenster,
Münster, Germany

Section 1

Training Models for Skull Base Surgery

Chapter 1

Training Models for Skull-Base and Vascular Micro-Neurosurgery

Uwe Spetzger, Julie Etingold and Andrej von Schilling

Abstract

This overview presents computer-based augmented reality (AR) and virtual reality (VR) tools, in-vitro and in-vivo models as useful teaching tools for neurosurgical training, especially in skull-base surgery. An easy set-up and practicable training model for ventricular drainage (VD) is demonstrated. The model allows to evaluate practices, pitfalls and traceability in a virtual but realistic set-up for simulating VD placement. Computer-assisted planning and simulation of skull-base approaches and integration within the daily neurosurgical routine with VR and AR models are discussed for neurosurgical education. A set-up for microvascular training on a plastic rat and a specific vascular anastomosis practice kit with different tube diameters of 1–3 mm of specific plastic vessels for the training of microvascular anastomoses is shown. End-to-end and end-to-side anastomoses were performed with different levels of difficulty, trying to simulate realistic conditions in bypass surgery. Additionally, the teaching strategy of experimental silicone aneurysm clipping in a 3D printed plastic skull and silicone brain model is demonstrated in video sequences. An experimental animal model with microsurgically created bifurcation aneurysms is discussed because this training model for clip occlusion of aneurysms on a living object, still has the greatest relevance to neurosurgical reality.

Keywords: neurosurgical training, experimental aneurysms, microvascular surgery, experimental surgical models, microsurgical training and education, in-vivo neurosurgical models, in-vitro neurosurgical models

1. Introduction

Today the younger neurosurgical generation has a reduced possibility for practical training in nearly all fields of neurosurgery. Accordingly, neurosurgical training models show increasing popularity. However, skull-base surgery often has a higher level of difficulty and is therefore rarely integrated into the basic surgical training of younger neurosurgeons. Even sophisticated modern, computer-based 3D models cannot adequately replace the important practical and hands-on surgical training. For this reason, we need realistic and gradually coordinated practical scenarios to learn and practice basic neurosurgical skills in sequential steps. Here we present some easy-to-implement practical examples that have proven themselves for operative training in skull-base surgery and for vascular microsurgery.

The number of skull-base procedures as well as microsurgical clipping of cerebral aneurysms is continuously decreasing. Meanwhile, the endovascular treatment of cerebral aneurysms has markedly reduced the number of microsurgical clipping procedures. The result will be a reduced possibility for practical training in aneurysm surgery, especially for the younger generation [1–3]. Stereotactic radiosurgery on one hand, and the increasing number of patients successfully treated by endovascular techniques on the other hand, will further reduce the overall caseload in skull-base and vascular microsurgery in the next years. However, especially huge, calcified or wide neck aneurysms will remain for microsurgical clip occlusion and will be a challenge for cerebrovascular neurosurgeons in the future. On the other hand, revascularisation and bypass techniques will be more and more in demand [4, 5]. Due to these conditions, concepts and realistic models for practical microsurgical training are necessary to improve the practical skills in neurosurgeons during their training, especially in the field of vascular and skull base surgery [6–12].

2. Computer-assisted training tools

2.1 Ventricular drainage (VD) model

Various VD training models have been developed, tested and published [13–15]. Recently, we performed another prospective study to evaluate practices, pitfalls and traceability in a realistic but virtual set-up for simulating ventricular drainage (VD) placement as a practicable training model using our navigation system (Brainlab, Munich, Germany), the navigation pointer functioning as a virtual VD catheter to be placed in the cMRI of a healthy subject (**Figure 1**). We evaluated accuracy by repeated virtual freehand VD placement on the prone subject using anatomical landmarks by neurosurgeons-in-training and non-neurosurgical staff. The influence of the level of neurosurgical knowledge and training level were of overall interest, especially in narrow ventricles. It was found that accurate VD placement correlated with neurosurgical experience (**Figures 2** and **3**). These initial results are not yet published, however.

This simple set-up is an easy model for continuous neurosurgical training, with the aim of optimizing the medical care of our patients and constantly improving the level of education. Its set-up could be varied further, for example, as a good training module for simulating an intraoperative emergency puncture of the ventricle, exemplary in an atypical pterional positioning of the head. This poses an unusual situation that requires high surgical skills with an excellent three-dimensional spatial concept.

2.2 Augmented reality (AR) and virtual reality (VR) training tools

Navigation systems offer a multitude of technical options that can be used for training and further education [16, 17]. Brainlab has been offering the function of transparent reflection in a superimposed display of previously segmented anatomical structures for over 20 years (**Figure 4**). This head-up display, as an early AR tool, in which the pre-planned and segmented structures are faded into the ocular of the operating microscope or onto the screen, allows optimal orientation and is didactically very valuable. However, the accusation is justified that we generally use these technical possibilities of virtual reality or augmented reality, offered as multiplanar visualization or as 3D reconstruction view, far too little for teaching and training purposes [17].

Recently, our department has been working with AR 3D models (UpSurgeOn S.r.l., Milan, Italy) to improve surgical and anatomical skills as well as presurgical positioning of the patient (**Figure 5**). For this, the department acquired partially reusable 3D models of the most common cranial neurosurgical approaches including certain pathologies (e.g., intracranial aneurysms) (**Figures 6–8**).

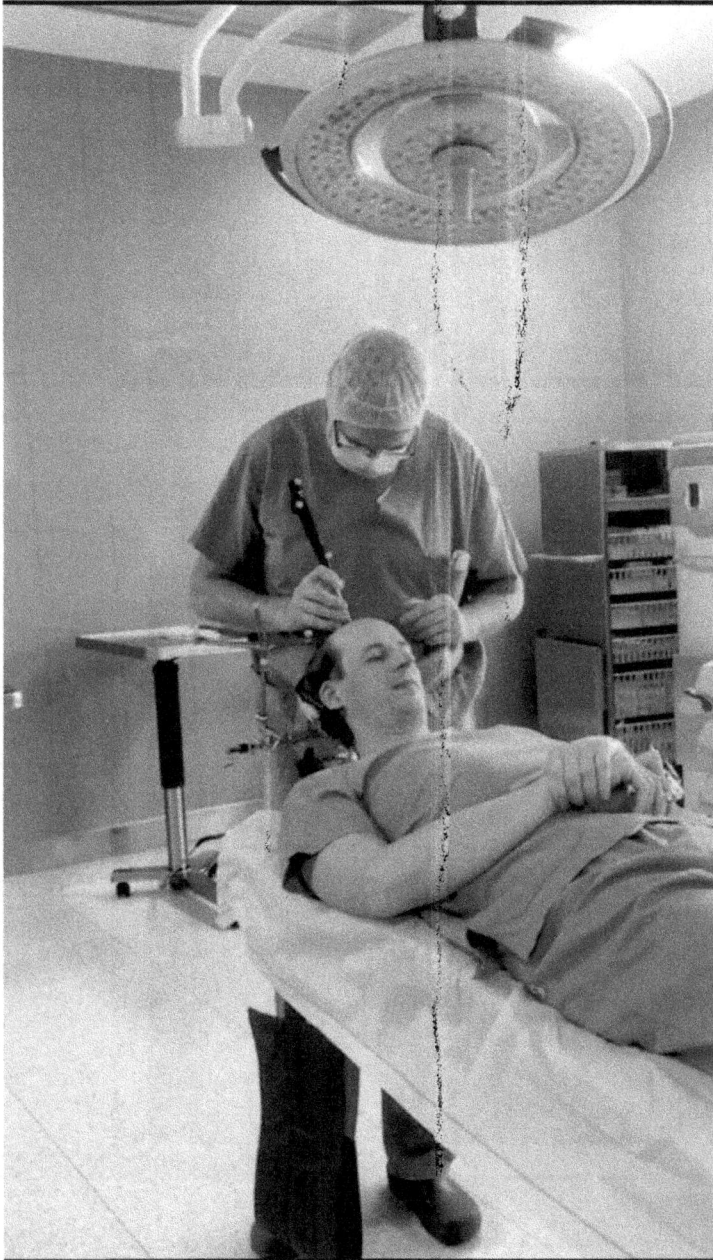

Figure 1.
Study set-up for virtual VD placement. The navigation pointer functions as a virtual VD catheter to be placed in the cMRI of a healthy subject.

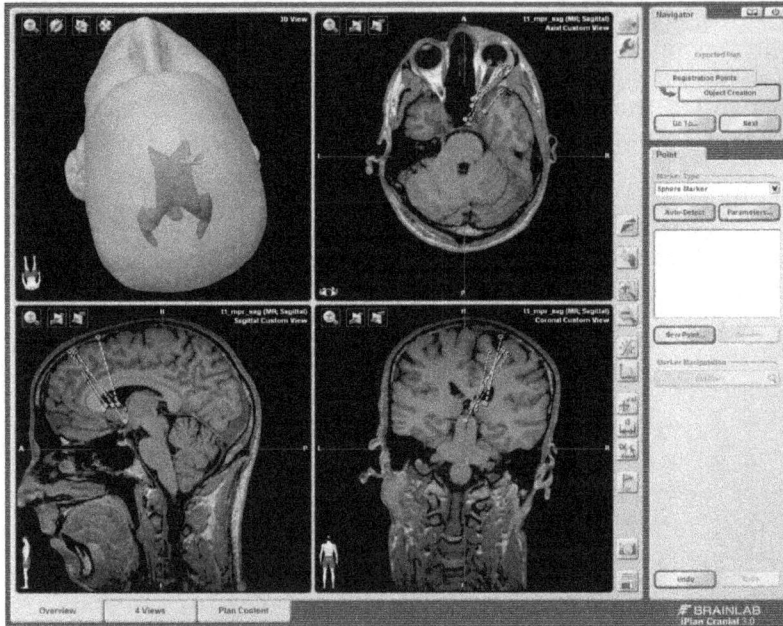

Figure 2.
A selection of virtual VD trajectories by participants with neurosurgical experience including the 'ideal trajectory' in blue.

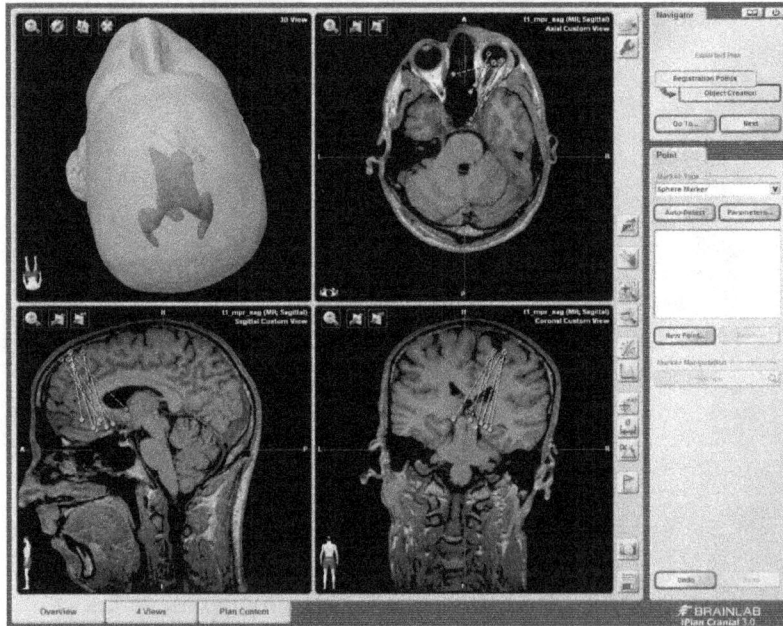

Figure 3.
A selection of virtual VD trajectories by participants without neurosurgical experience including the 'ideal trajectory' in blue.

The 3D models are made of synthetic materials which render them extremely lifelike in haptics and handling. They can be used as are or in conjunction with an AR app (UpSurgeOn Neurosurgery S.r.l., Milan, Italy), which walks

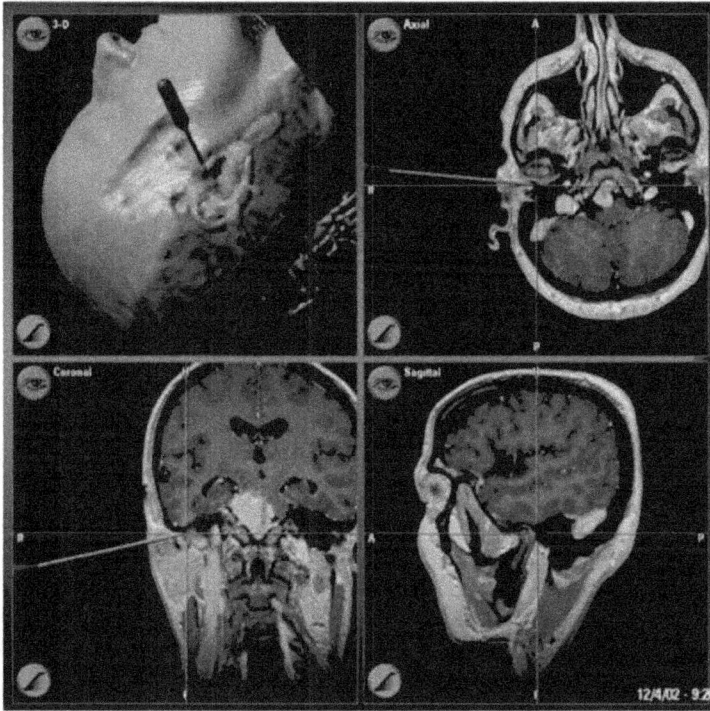

Figure 4.
Intraoperative screenshot during a skull base procedure performed on April 12, 2002, shows then state-of-the-art technology with intraoperative AR tools that were already available at the time. The preoperatively segmented relevant anatomical structures are demonstrated and the navigation pointer shows the trajectory to the clival meningioma via a combined antero-sigmoidal/sub-temporal approach. The dominant sigmoid and transverse sinus (green) and the lateralized basilar artery (magenta) displaced by the tumor are visualized.

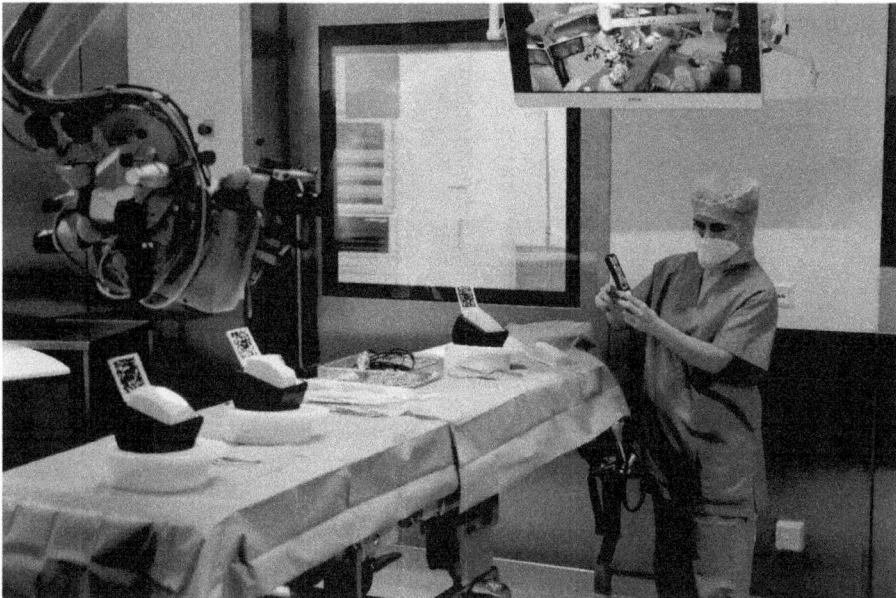

Figure 5.
Our setup for a cadaver-free manual training session with AR 3D models (UpSurgeOn S.r.l., Milan, Italy).

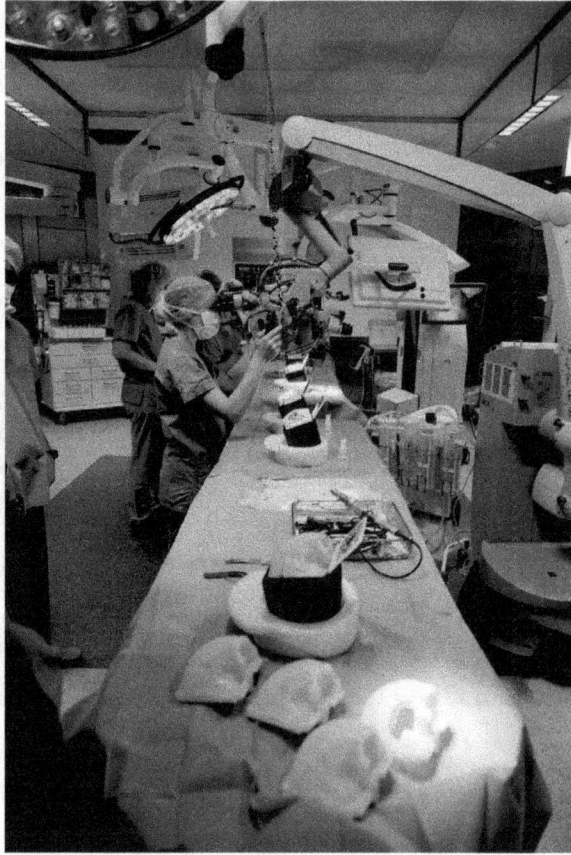

Figure 6.
Our setup for a cadaver-free manual training session with AR 3D models (UpSurgeOn S.r.l., Milan, Italy). The models can be reused by purchasing additional craniotomy covers as depicted here.

the surgeon through the entire procedure by fusing a virtual image with the actual model, starting with optimal positioning of the patient for the specific surgery (**Figures 9–11**). The app also allows an image of the patient awaiting the planned procedure to be projected into any space, allowing the surgeon a 360° view. Training sessions were held for neurosurgery residents, offering them the opportunity to practice neurosurgical approaches safely, including craniotomies, drilling with various bits, brain retraction, basic intradural dissection and even aneurysm clip placement. We acquired a navigational data set for one of the models by placing it in a CT-scanner and uploading the data set it into our navigation system (Brainlab, Munich, Germany), thereby giving participants the additional chance to practice the procedure image-guided in a non-bloody and risk-free manner whilst getting more familiar with the navigation system itself (**Figure 12**). Our results concerning the efficacy of this kind of modern training model have yet to be published; however, anecdotally, residents report feeling more secure in their surgical approaches, in choosing and handling surgical drills as well as in the positioning of patients for surgery. Some residents now use the UpSurgeOn App to plan surgeries in advance or to double-check the preoperative positioning of the patient by overlaying the actual patient with an AR model.

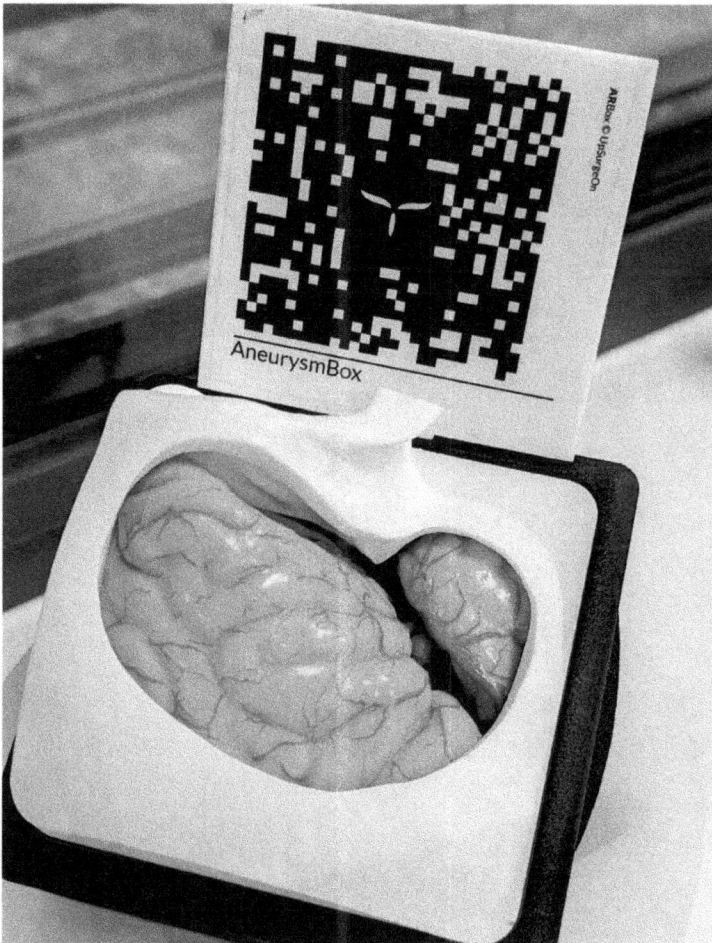

Figure 7.
Close-up of the 'aneurysm box' including the craniotomy model, the synthetic brain and vessels and the associated QR code for use in conjunction with the Upsurgeon App for an AR component. The right-sided aneurysm is partially visible through the Sylvian fissure.

Due to the relative ease and cost-effectiveness of implementing the aforementioned tools, we consider simulation-based cadaver-free training with AR a promising option to bring skull-base surgery training to a new level.

The intense occupation with radiological images, necessary for the segmentation of a tumour or any other lesion and the marking of the anatomical structures, already brings great didactic benefit to the colleagues who are in training. During surgery, the recognition value of the anatomical structures rendered in the CT or MRT as a three-dimensional surgical site under the surgical microscope provides the greatest learning value. The use of navigation data for the dedicated operation planning and the daily discussion of the surgical cases are essential for this. Particularly, in the case of complex skull base operations, the position, craniotomy, microsurgical strategy and resulting operation-specific risks should routinely be discussed with the assistant physicians on the day before the surgical procedure in a pre-op conference. In particular, the discussion of surgery-specific anatomy on the basis of the 3D navigation data provides optimal preparation for

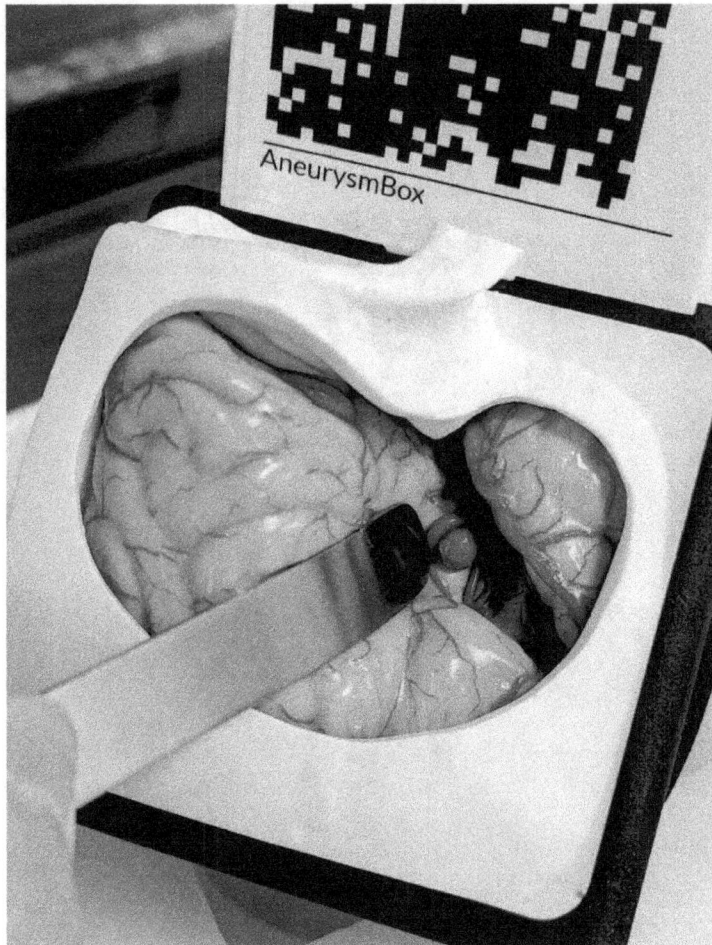

Figure 8.
Retracting the synthetic brain to expose the right-sided MCA aneurysm. The materials used render the models extremely lifelike in haptics and handling.

these complex neurosurgical interventions [17]. So the following day, the display of the operation-specific anatomical structures via the head-up display during surgery will provide a much higher didactic benefit for complex skull base procedures (**Figure 13**).

3. In-vitro microsurgical models

Here we present two sophisticated in-vitro artificial plastic models which closely mimic real vascular conditions and a more complex in-vivo experimental animal bifurcation aneurysm model in rabbits [18]. For initial and basic microvascular training, the poly-vinyl-chloride (PVC) rat model (Microsurgical Developments Foundation, Maastricht, The Netherlands) shows itself to be more or less sufficient [19]. For a more realistic haptic feeling and enhanced specific microvascular training, a model with highly elastic polyvinyl alcohol (PVA) vessels and an anatomical plastic head (Kezlex, Ono & Co., Ltd., Tokyo, Japan) is available [18, 20].

Figure 9.
The models can be used as are or in conjunction with an AR app (UpSurgeOn Neurosurgery S.r.l., Milan, Italy) via a QR code as pictured here. The materials used render the models extremely lifelike in haptics and handling. Depicted here is a right-sided pterional approach with craniotomy already performed. The underlying synthetic dura is visible.

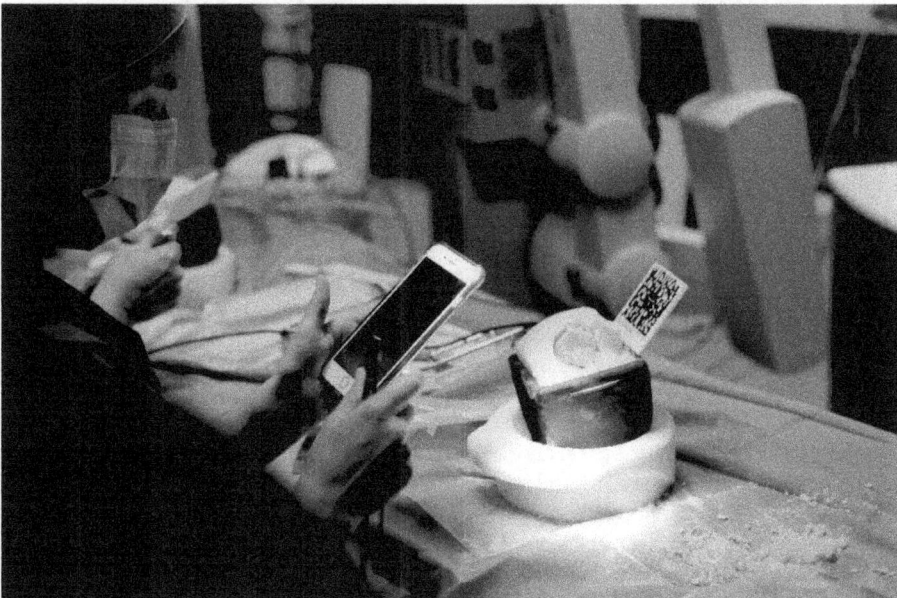

Figure 10.
Here the 3D model is fused with a virtual image via the accompanying QR code, allowing the surgeon to explore deeper intracranial structures of the specific surgical approach.

Additionally, our highly sophisticated in-vivo experimental animal model (rabbit carotid artery bifurcation model) is demonstrated and discussed [21–23].

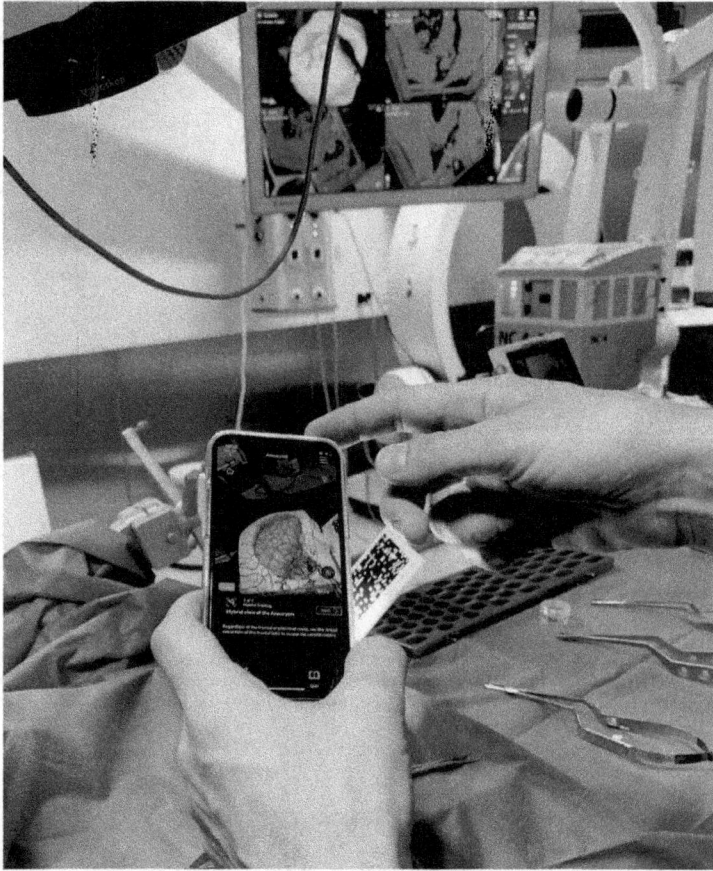

Figure 11.
Hybrid view of one of the 3D models showing a right-sided ICA aneurysm.

3.1 PVC rat model

Using the PVC rat model for 'unbloody training' of microsurgical techniques and improvement of practical skills is a perfect example of the replacement of living animals (**Figure 14**). The number of live animals used for in-vivo training will likely be reduced in the future, therefore these in-vitro methods will be needed to make the transition to in-vivo models easier. The PVC rat model (Microsurgical Developments Foundation, Maastricht, The Netherlands) should be the first step in the practical education and allow various microsurgical training situations. The replacement of the plastic vessels is easy and relatively cheap [19]. Using a specific nozzle at the back of the rat model, the colored vessels can be filled with water, thus permitting an easy check of patency and quality of the anastomosis.

In the prospective part of our published study [18], end-to-end and end-to-side anastomoses were performed with three different levels of difficulty in the PVC rat model. In total six surgeons with different expertises and different levels of vascular training and surgical skills performed these microsurgical procedures. Different sizes of plastic tubes of various lengths and diameters were used for reduction of the surgical approach and the workspace, to adapt the experimental set-up to a scenario with different degrees of difficulty (**Figure 15**). Those plastic tubes reduce the operative field and consecutively the surgical working space and determine the trajectory and

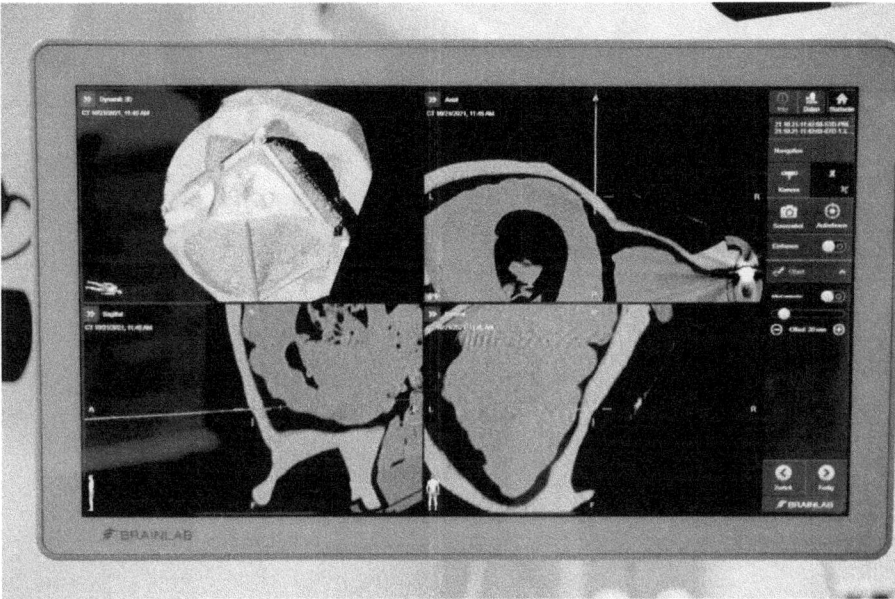

Figure 12.
The navigational data set for the 3D model of an MCA aneurysm.

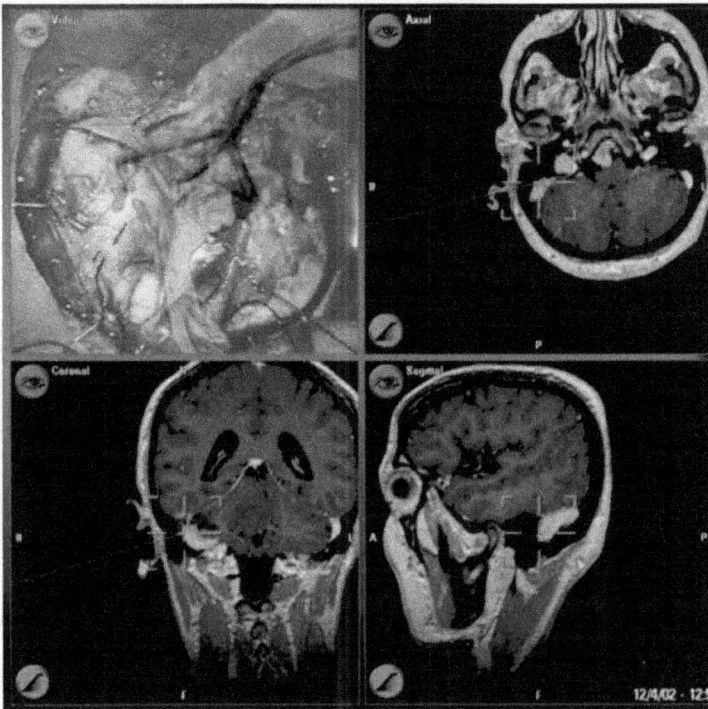

Figure 13.
The operating microscope (Neuro NC4, Carl Zeiss) was linked and registered with the navigation system (Brainlab VectorVision). After the combined craniotomy and opening of the dura, AR overlay head-up display depicts the dominant sigmoid and transverse sinus (green), the basilar artery (magenta) and the clival meningioma below.

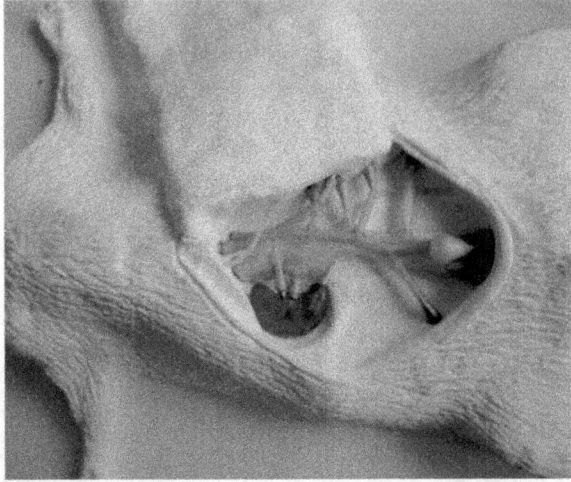

Figure 14.
In-vitro model with plastic vessels of the abdominal cavity of the PVC rat (Microsurgical Developments Foundation, Maastricht, The Netherlands).

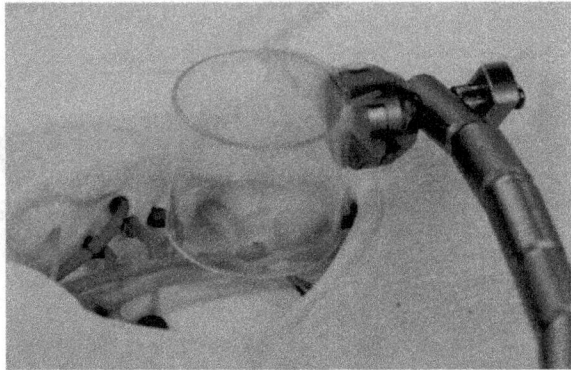

Figure 15.
A transparent plastic tube was brought into the operative field and fixed to a conventional flexible retractor system to reduce the working space and mimic surgical conditions in deeper approaches. In this narrow workspace, the level of difficulty to perform an anastomosis significantly increases.

the direction for the instruments. Due to this focused working channel, the degree of freedom for using the instruments is restricted and therefore, the level of difficulty to perform an adequate anastomosis increases significantly (**Figure 15**). The different sizes of the plastic tubes mimic intraoperative conditions in a narrow and deep surgical field. Plastic tube I (Advanced) has a diameter of 40 mm and a depth of 15 mm. Tube II (Expert) has a diameter of 30 mm and a depth of 35 mm (**Figure 15**). Tube III (Master) has a diameter of 25 mm and a depth of 45 mm. For the anastomoses, we used conventional microsurgical instruments and monofile polyamid sutures 8/0 (BV 2 needle), respectively, 10/0 (BV 100-4 needle) Ethilon (Ethicon, Johnson & Johnson MEDICAL GmbH, Norderstedt, Germany).

In this experimental set-up, the increase of surgical complexity by reducing the workspace with the different plastic tubes clearly demonstrates that the time of surgery to perform the anastomosis increased significantly (**Figure 15**). In addition, the rate of incorrect sutures of the vessel wall increased, the narrower the surgical field

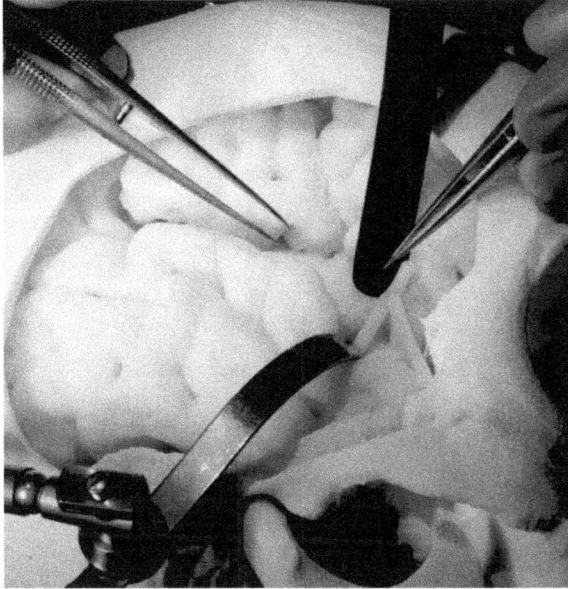

Figure 16.
This plastic skull and silicone brain model shows an extended pterional approach with slight retraction and opening of the Sylvian fissure. An end-to-side anastomosis was performed using highly elastic PVA-vessels (Kezlex, Ono & Co., Ltd., Tokyo, Japan). This set-up allows for a realistic scenario and the handling of the vessels during the anastomosis, closely mimicking human conditions during bypass surgery.

became due to the decreasing diameter of the tube. Therefore, the overall patency rate of the anastomosis was clearly reduced with increasing grade of complexity [18].

3.2 PVA vessel with craniotomy site

The wet PVA vessels of the vascular anastomosis practice kit are transparent, highly flexible and soft [20]. However, they have to be kept moist and tend to dry out and lose their elasticity, especially under the high-energy xenon light of the operating microscope. At present, we have used the PVA vessels of the vascular anastomosis practice kit for various experimental anastomoses. Compared to the PVC vessels in the rat model, the preparation and handling of the PVA vessels, especially the grasping with a forceps or the insertion of the needle into the vessel wall is much more realistic and closely mimics human conditions.

An even more realistic scenario is provided by the plastic skull model with relatively soft and deformable silicone brain material and the vascular anastomosis practice kit with highly elastic plastic (PVA) vessels (Kezlex, Ono & Co., Ltd., Tokyo, Japan). The very soft and elastic plastic vessels of the vascular anastomosis practice kit are available in three different diameters: 1 mm, 2 mm and 3 mm. The vascular kit with the humid PVA vessels has a perfect haptic feeling during preparation, cutting and suturing of the vessels. The whole set-up with the deformable plastic brain, the realistic feeling of retraction and especially the optical impression under the microscope generate an overall aspect of a real microsurgical scenario closely mimicking human conditions.

The 3D model with pterional craniotomy and the deformable frontal and temporal lobe (Kezlex, Ono & Co., Ltd., Tokyo, Japan) is a perfect in-vitro model to simulate an opened Sylvian fissure for experimental bypass, as well as aneurysm surgery training.

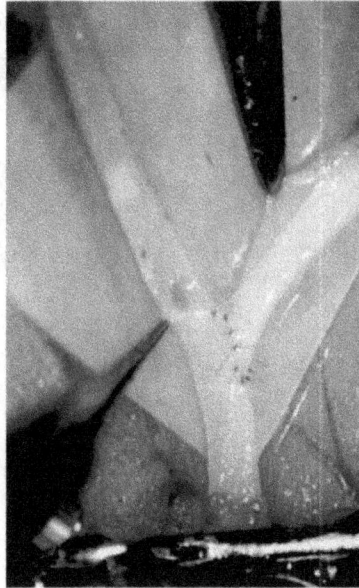

Figure 17.
In-vitro model in a rabbit. An end-to-side anastomosis of both carotid arteries was created using 10/0 sutures to generate an arterial bifurcation.

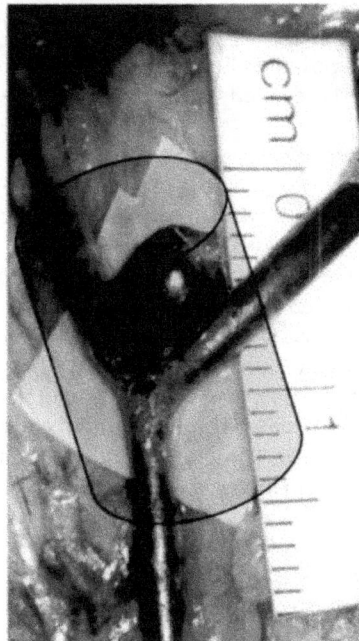

Figure 18.
The insertion of a venous pouch into the bifurcation finally results in an experimental bifurcation aneurysm, comparable to a 6 mm MCA aneurysm with a broad neck. The in-vivo bifurcation aneurysm model is a perfect training tool for clip application, especially if a plastic tube (schematic drawing) creates a narrow workspace with limited access for the clip applicator. Due to the determined trajectory, the clip occlusion of the aneurysm mimics human conditions. This set-up is a sophisticated in-vivo training model for active teaching and practical training for bypass surgery, as well as aneurysm clipping.

This set-up allows a realistic retraction of the Sylvian fissure, its handling and preparation closely imitating human conditions (**Figure 16**).

We also used 3D printed aneurysms made from soft PVA tubing that could be clipped for training purposes. The 3D printed hollow aneurysms were positioned in the depth of the Sylvian fissure and so microsurgical clip application could be simulated adequately (Videos 1 and 2, https://bit.ly/3AeRgNk). Then the experimental plastic aneurysm could be removed from the site to assess the success of the clipping maneuver (Video 3, https://bit.ly/3AeRgNk). These realistic human skull and brain models are relatively expensive but could be used repeatedly [24, 25]. If the models are integrated into practical teaching and training, they help to establish a realistic microsurgical scenario and are definitively superior to computer-based animations alone [26].

4. In-vivo microsurgical models

4.1 Rabbit model for experimental bifurcation aneurysms

The materials and methods of the experimental aneurysm bifurcation model in rabbits (**Figure 17**) were described in great detail in previous publications [21–23]. The developed and previously described animal bifurcation aneurysm model is a perfect and highly realistic vivisection model for education and practical training for microsurgical handling and preparation of cerebral vessels. However, this model should be used as a final education tool in an advanced stage of training. The blood flow, the vessel diameter, the haptic feedback, even the induced vasospasms by manipulating too roughly, and the tension of the vessel walls, all of this can be compared to vascular microsurgery in humans (**Figures 17** and **18**). Therefore, it is an optimal training tool for all cerebrovascular reconstructive surgical procedures and maintains expert status in bypass surgery [27].

Additionally, this experimental aneurysm model allows an optimal practical training of clip application and is a realistic teaching model for optimizing clip occlusion of cerebral aneurysms. As described in the PVC rat model study conditions, the different sizes of plastic tubes were also integrated into our experimental animal model (**Figure 18**). The tubes were fixed to a conventional and flexible retractor system and could be removed easily if difficulties arise, especially inadvertent bleeding intraoperatively. The transparent plastic tubes create a narrow and deep surgical approach by restricting the angle of view and determining the trajectory of the clip occlusion of the aneurysm as in real aneurysm surgery. After clipping of the experimental bifurcation aneurysm, the plastic tube was removed and the aneurysm could be inspected easily from all sides and the clip position could be checked adequately.

For repeated training, the clip was removed from the experimental aneurysm and the procedure could be repeated, for example, with a narrower, longer or differently angled plastic tube, creating a completely new situation with a different view and access to the experimental bifurcation aneurysm. This high-end in-vitro animal model is an excellent and realistic set-up for intensive practical training and teaching of aneurysm clipping. However, it takes a great deal of logistical and technical effort to produce such an experimental animal aneurysm.

5. Conclusion

VR and AR are currently established in many areas of medical education and should increasingly become the standard in modern neurosurgical advanced teaching and training as well. Therefore, these tools should also be used regularly for surgical training and further education of young neurosurgeons. With modern navigation systems, diverse software and hardware components are generally available and should consequently be used and strictly integrated into our daily clinical routine. This technology thus forms the basis for highly qualified practical training in skull base surgery. In addition, it facilitates the necessary interdisciplinary cooperation between faculties and offers the opportunity for lifelong learning for all surgically active colleagues in skull base surgery.

In-vitro models, like the AR 3D models, the PVC rat model or the PVA vascular model combined with the realistic brain and craniotomy site, allow for a perfect set-up for the advanced training of microsurgery and microvascular anastomoses. The main advantages of these artificial plastic models are their overall availability, the low price and the lack of a specific OR set-up or instruments, compared to training in in-vivo models. The costs and logistical considerations, as well as the ethical and legal aspects involved in maintaining living animals for education and training, make in-vivo models a relatively impractical tool.

These in-vitro models are easily adaptable to the respective circumstances and allow unhindered practical training under almost realistic operating conditions. The surgical complexity with end-to-end and end-to-side anastomoses could be adapted in models and the success rate is easy to check. Parameters like the time of surgery, the rate of incorrect sutures of the vessel wall and the overall patency rate of the anastomoses can be clearly monitored, as well as the learning curve. Therefore, these in-vitro models form the basis for the first step in basic practical training and are a prerequisite for a successful career in vascular neurosurgery and skull base surgery.

In-vivo models should be the last step of practical education. Like our experimental animal model with the insertion of a venous pouch within the microsurgically created arterial bifurcation represents an advanced training model very close to realistic human conditions. In the first step of this model, microvascular anastomoses are trained and secondly, the resulting bifurcation aneurysm is a perfect training tool to learn clip application. Especially, if a plastic tube is positioned over the surgical field and creates a narrow approach with restricted workspace and limited scope for manipulation for the correct clip occlusion of the aneurysm. Our experimental animal model represents a higher level of surgical vascular expertise and additionally is a perfect model to practice bypass surgery, as well as the appropriate handling of clip application and clip occlusion of cerebral aneurysms.

Conflict of interest

The authors have no financial relationship with the organizations mentioned in the paper. All authors declare that they have no conflict of interest.

Author details

Uwe Spetzger[1,2]*, Julie Etingold[1] and Andrej von Schilling[1]

1 Department of Neurosurgery, Klinikum Karlsruhe, Karlsruhe, Germany

2 Institute for Anthropomatics and Robotics, Humanoids and Intelligence System Lab, Karlsruhe Institute of Technology, KIT, Karlsruhe, Germany

*Address all correspondence to: uwe.spetzger@klinikum-karlsruhe.de

IntechOpen

References

[1] Mori K, Yamamoto T, Nakao Y, Esaki TMori K, Yamamoto T, Nakao Y, et al. Development of artificial cranial base model with soft tissues for practical education: Technical note. Neurosurgery. 2010;**66**(6 Suppl Operative):339-341; discussion 341. DOI: 10.1227/01. neu.0000369664.24998.b6

[2] Aboud E, Al-Mefty O, Yaşargil MG. New laboratory model for neurosurgical training that simulates live surgery. Journal of Neurosurgery. 2002;**97**(6): 1367-1372. DOI: 10.3171/jns.2002.97.6. 1367

[3] Gailloud P, Pray JR, Muster M, Piotin M, Fasel JH, Rüfenacht DA. An in vitro anatomic model of the human cerebral arteries with saccular arterial aneurysms. Surgical and Radiologic Anatomy. 1997;**19**(2):119-121

[4] Gruber A, Bavinszki G, Killer M, Al Shameri A, Richling B. In vitro training model for endovascular embolization of cerebral aneurysms. Minimally Invasive Neurosurgery. 1997;**40**(4):121-123. DOI: 10.1055/s-2008-1053431

[5] Senior MA, Southern SJ, Majumder S. Microvascular simulator—a device for micro-anastomosis training. Annals of the Royal College of Surgeons of England. 2001;**83**(5):358-360

[6] Colpan ME, Slavin KV, Amin-Hanjani S, Calderon-Arnuphi M, Charbel FT. Microvascular anastomosis training model based on a turkey neck with perfused arteries. Neurosurgery. 2008;**62**(5 Suppl. 2):ONS407-10; discussion ONS410-1. DOI: 10.1227/01. neu.0000326026.01349.75

[7] Hicdonmez T, Hamamcioglu MK, Tiryaki M, Cukur Z, Cobanoglu S. Microneurosurgical training model in fresh cadaveric cow brain: A laboratory study simulating the approach to the circle of Willis. Surgical Neurology. 2006;**66**(1):100-104; discussion 104. DOI: 10.1016/j.surneu.2005.09.027

[8] Hino A. Training in microvascular surgery using a chicken wing artery. Neurosurgery. 2003;**52**(6):1495-1497; discussion 1497-1498. DOI: 10.1227/01. neu.0000065174.83840.62

[9] Olabe J, Olabe J, Roda JM, Sancho V. Human cadaver brain infusion skull model for neurosurgical training. Surgical Neurology International. 2011;**2**:54. DOI: 10.4103/2152-7806.80119. Epub 2011 Apr 28

[10] Giovani A, Sandu AM, Petrescu G, Gorgan RM, Goel A. Application of microanastomosis techniques in vascular neurosurgery training and innovation of future surgical strategies for giant aneurysms. World Neurosurgery. 2019;**122**:e1120-e1127. DOI: 10.1016/j.wneu.2018.10.239. Epub 2018 Nov 12

[11] Scholz M, Mücke T, Düring MV, Pechlivanis I, Schmieder K, Harders AG. Microsurgically induced aneurysm models in rats, part I: Techniques and histological examination. Minimally Invasive Neurosurgery. 2008;**51**(2): 76-82. DOI: 10.1055/s-2008-1058088

[12] Tellioglu AT, Eker E, Cimen K, Comert A, Karaeminogullari G, Tekdemir I. Training model for microvascular anastomosis. The Journal of Craniofacial Surgery. 2009;**20**(1):238-239. DOI: 10.1097/SCS.0b013e318 1843ade

[13] Krombach G, Ganser A, Fricke C, Rohde V, Reinges M, Gilsbach J, et al. Virtual placement of frontal ventricular catheters using frameless neuronavigation: An "unbloody training" for young neurosurgeons. Minimally Invasive Neurosurgery.

2000;**43**(4):171-175. DOI: 10.1055/
s-2000-11376

[14] Perin A, Galbiati TF, Gambatesa E, Ayadi R, Orena EF, Cuomo V, et al. Filling the gap between the OR and virtual simulation: A European study on a basic neurosurgical procedure. Acta Neurochirurgica. 2018;**160**(11):2087-2097. DOI: 10.1007/s00701-018-3676-8. Epub 2018 Oct 1

[15] Tai BL, Rooney D, Stephenson F, Liao PS, Sagher O, Shih AJ, et al. Development of a 3D-printed external ventricular drain placement simulator: Technical note. Journal of Neurosurgery. 2015;**123**(4):1070-1076. DOI: 10.3171/2014.12.JNS141867. Epub 2015 Jun 26

[16] Spetzger U, Laborde G, Gilsbach JM. Frameless neuronavigation in modern neurosurgery. Minimally Invasive Neurosurgery. 1995;**38**(4):163-166. DOI: 10.1055/s-2008-1053478

[17] König A, Spetzger U, editors. Surgery of the Skull Base. Practical Diagnosis and Therapy. Springer International Publishing; 2018. DOI: 10.1007/978-3-319-64018-1

[18] Spetzger U, von Schilling A, Brombach T, Winkler G. Training models for vascular microneurosurgery. Acta Neurochirurgica. Supplement. 2011;**112**:115-119. DOI: 10.1007/978-3-7091-0661-7_21

[19] Remie R. The PVC-rat and other alternatives in microsurgical training. Lab Animal (NY). 2001;**30**(9):48-52. DOI: 10.1038/5000109

[20] Mutoh T, Ishikawa T, Ono H, Yasui N. A new polyvinyl alcohol hydrogel vascular model (KEZLEX) for microvascular anastomosis training. Surgical Neurology International. 2010;**1**:74. DOI: 10.4103/2152-7806. 72626

[21] Spetzger U, Reul J, Weis J, Bertalanffy H, Thron A, Gilsbach JM. Microsurgically produced bifurcation aneurysms in a rabbit model for endovascular coil embolization. Journal of Neurosurgery. 1996;**85**(3):488-495. DOI: 10.3171/jns.1996.85.3.0488

[22] Reul J, Spetzger U, Weis J, Sure U, Gilsbach JM, Thron A. Endovascular occlusion of experimental aneurysms with detachable coils: Influence of packing density and perioperative anticoagulation. Neurosurgery. 1997;**41**(5):1160-1165; discussion 1165-1168. DOI: 10.1097/00006123-199711000-00028

[23] Spetzger U, Reul J, Weis J, Bertalanffy H, Gilsbach JM. Endovascular coil embolization of microsurgically produced experimental bifurcation aneurysms in rabbits. Surgical Neurology. 1998;**49**(5):491-494. DOI: 10.1016/s0090-3019(96) 00437-5

[24] Mashiko T, Kaneko N, Konno T, Otani K, Nagayama R, Watanabe E. Training in cerebral aneurysm clipping using self-made 3-dimensional models. Journal of Surgical Education. 2017;**74**(4):681-689. DOI: 10.1016/j. jsurg.2016.12.010. Epub 2017 Jan 16

[25] Błaszczyk M, Jabbar R, Szmyd B, Radek M. 3D printing of rapid, low-cost and patient-specific models of brain vasculature for use in preoperative planning in clipping of intracranial aneurysms. Journal of Clinical Medicine. 2021;**10**(6):1201. DOI: 10.3390/jcm10061201

[26] Kimura Y, Mashiko T, Watanabe E, Kawai K. Preoperative simulation of a middle cerebral artery aneurysm clipping using a rotational three-dimensional digital subtraction angiography. Surgical Neurology International. 2021;**12**:70. DOI: 10.25259/SNI_934_2020

[27] Tantongtip D, Fratianni A, Jenkner J, Arnold S, Spetzger U. Surgical treatment of inadvertent internal carotid artery lesion by extra-intracranial high-flow bypass. A case report and review of the literature. Journal of Neurological Surgery Reports. 2015;76(1):e100-e104. DOI: 10.1055/s-0035-1551670. Epub 2015 May 15

Section 2

Radiotherapy

Chapter 2

Stereotactic Radiotherapy for Benign Skull Base Tumors

Arnar Astradsson

Abstract

Benign skull base tumors include meningiomas, pituitary adenomas, craniopharyngiomas, and vestibular schwannomas. As an adjuvant therapy to surgery or when surgical treatment carries too high a risk of complications, a highly precise focused radiation, known as stereotactic radiosurgery or fractionated stereotactic radiation therapy, can be delivered to the tumor. The aim of this chapter is to systematically discuss benefits of the therapy, i.e., tumor control as well as complications and risk factors of the therapy relating to vision, hearing, hormone secreting regions, and cerebral vasculature. Meningiomas, pituitary adenomas, craniopharyngiomas, and vestibular schwannomas constitute the majority of primary skull base tumors amenable to stereotactic radiation therapy or radiosurgery and will be described in this chapter.

Keywords: skull base tumors, stereotactic radiosurgery, fractionated stereotactic radiotherapy, tumor control, vision, hearing, hormonal, stroke

1. Introduction

Stereotactic radiosurgery (SRS) is defined as a single application of a high dose of radiation to a stereotactically precisely defined target [1, 2]. Stereotactic radiosurgery of the brain using the Gamma Knife or a Linear accelerator (LINAC) is a well-established and very effective therapy for brain metastases, arteriovenous malformations, and benign skull base tumors [1, 2]. The treatment utilizes differences in the biological sensitivity and repair capability of normal and pathologic tissue [3]. Stereotactic principles are used for calculating the radiation field. The patient wears a stereotactic head frame and undergoes a computed tomography (CT), which is subsequently fused with a preexisting magnetic resonance (MRI) scan, or an MRI is performed in the stereotactic head frame, the disadvantage being that there are often distortions of the magnetic field [4]. However, most lesions are better demonstrated on MRI scans. The aim of dose planning is to deliver a maximal dose to the tumor, while minimizing radiation dose to healthy brain structures. This is accomplished with conforming the radiation to the target and applying steep dose gradients [1, 2].

LINAC-based radiosurgery and radiation therapy devices accelerate electrons, and the electron beam is aimed at a heavy metal alloy target [1]. The resulting interactions between the electrons and the target produce photons, which can be collimated and focused on a patient. Multiple radiation beams are applied, each of which has its own entrance and exit points, while all are directed at the same target where they cross each other [1]. In LINAC radiosurgery and fractionated radiation therapy, both the gantry and the treatment table rotate around the isocenter of the lesion for accurate delivery of the multiple beams [1]. The single radiosurgery radiation dose prescribed in LINAC-based radiosurgery for benign skull base tumors is commonly 10–17.5 Gy [1, 4–6]. Notably, in case of lesions adjacent to radiosensitive structures, fractionation is the preferred method of delivery, in which case different dose regimes apply [1, 7, 8]. In contrast to the Gamma Knife, LINAC offers the option of dose fractionation. Fractionated stereotactic radiation therapy (FSRT) utilizes the principles of conventional fractionation while taking advantage of stereotactic dosimetric techniques to conform the radiation to the tumor target. It is particularly suitable for treating skull base tumors, close to eloquent structures, such as the pituitary gland and optic nerves. A commonly used prescription dose for benign skull base tumors is a total of 54 Gy given with 1.8–2.0 Gy per fraction.

Radiosurgery with the Gamma Knife uses 201 separate cobalt sources, all aimed at a high dose at precisely one fixed target, with one or more isocenters employed, depending on the size and shape of the tumor [1–3]. A commonly used dose for benign skull base tumors is 12 Gy–16 Gy [3, 9].

Cyberknife is used in some centers and is a frameless robotic radiosurgery system, which is typically delivered in multiple session. It is a relatively safe and effective treatment for skull base tumors [10].

More recently, proton beam therapy has been introduced and is gaining progressively widespread use. It relies on protons produced end emitted by a synchrotron or cyclotron. The protons travel to a specific depth in the body depending on their energy and when striking the tumor rapidly emit their energy. It is well suited and used for various benign skull base tumors. Proton beam therapy is an effective treatment modality, with favorable long-term tumor control rates [11, 12].

The differences between Gamma Knife, LINAC and Cyberknife are summarized in **Table 1**.

	Gamma knife	**LINAC**	**Cyberknife**
Use	Developed exclusively for brain surgery	Not developed exclusively for brain surgery	Developed primarily for brain surgery but can be used for other regions
Accuracy	Millimeter accuracy	Millimeter accuracy	Submillimeter accuracy
Irradiation source	Gamma rays from Cobalt-60 source	6-MV X-rays	Compact linac with 6 MeV photons
Beam arrangements	201 fixed concentric non-opposed beams	Non-coplanar arcs • Dynamic arc rotation • Conical rotation - Static beam arrangements	Robotic arm with 6 degrees of freedom of movement; nonisocentric, where beams can be directed from any desired angle
Head fixation	A lightweight stereotactic frame is affixed to the head for rigid stabilization	Thermoplastic face mask, less rigid	Does not need head fixation, thus more flexible
Number of treatment sessions	Single treatment session	Single or multiple (i.e., 30) treatment sessions	Single or multiple (hypofractionated) up to five treatment sessions

Table 1.
Differences between gamma knife, LINAC, and cyberknife.

2. Stereotactic radiosurgery and fractionated stereotactic radiation therapy of benign skull base tumors

Meningiomas, pituitary adenomas, craniopharyngiomas, and vestibular schwannomas constitute the vast majority of primary skull base tumors suitable for stereotactic radiation therapy or radiosurgery.

2.1 Meningiomas

Meningiomas are the most common primary intracranial tumors, the prevalence being approximately 100 per 100,000 [13, 14]. They are slow-growing tumors, most often benign and dural-based. Meningiomas are classified according to the World Health Organization (WHO) classification of grade, where grade I is benign, grade II atypical, and grade III anaplastic [13, 15–17]. Approximately 95% of intracranial meningiomas are benign and approximately 5% are atypical or anaplastic [13, 15]. Atypical and anaplastic meningiomas have an increased recurrence and mortality risk [15, 16]. In addition to WHO grade, prognosis and recurrence risk depend on the radicality of resection [13, 18]. Anterior skull base meningiomas are defined as arising anterior to the chiasmatic sulcus, which separates the middle and the anterior cranial fossa. Anterior skull base meningiomas include olfactory groove, tuberculum sellae, sphenoid wing, cavernous sinus, and optic nerve sheath meningiomas [19, 20]. Medial skull base meningiomas include clival and petroclival meningiomas [21]. Olfactory groove meningiomas arise from the cribriform plate in the midline and often compress or distort the olfactory and optic nerves and optic chiasm (**Figure 1**). Tuberculum sellae meningiomas are usually located in the suprasellar and subchiasmal region in the midline and often compress the optic nerves and internal carotid arteries (**Figure 2**). Sphenoid wing meningiomas arise from the sphenoid wing and often involve the optic nerves, the cavernous sinus, or carotid arteries, and cause neurological damage by direct compression of adjacent cranial nerves (**Figure 3**). Cavernous sinus meningiomas may either originate within the cavernous sinus and spread outside of it or originate outside the cavernous sinus and invade it. Cavernous sinus meningiomas often present with symptoms related to compression of structures within the cavernous sinus, resulting in ophthalmoplegia or facial pain or numbness or ischemic stroke due to compression of the carotid artery and with tumor extending beyond the cavernous sinus, can also affect the optic nerves and chiasm or the pituitary gland (**Figure 4**). Total resection is often not possible, and resection is also associated with risks to the carotid artery, or damage to the cranial nerves of the cavernous sinus [22]. Optic nerve sheath meningiomas are rare, accounting for 1–2% of intracranial meningiomas, and due to their localization, management is often conservative. Finally, clival and petroclival meningiomas arise from the clivus and typically compress the brain stem, and they often involve the cavernous sinus and are surgically particularly challenging (**Figure 5**) [21].

With incompletely resected or recurrent skull base meningiomas, stereotactic radiation therapy or radiosurgery is recommended [13, 23]. Also, the extent of surgical tumor removal is dependent on tumor's localization adjacent to critical structures. Surgical treatment of cavernous sinus meningiomas, in particular, is associated with a high risk of cranial nerve injury, especially ophthalmoplegia, and therefore a high proportion of cavernous sinus meningiomas are treated by stereotactic radiation or radiosurgery and in some institutions is the first-line treatment. Generally, stereotactic radiosurgery or fractionated radiation therapy is frequently used as primary therapy in surgically high-risk tumors, resulting in good local control [4, 10, 13, 23, 24].

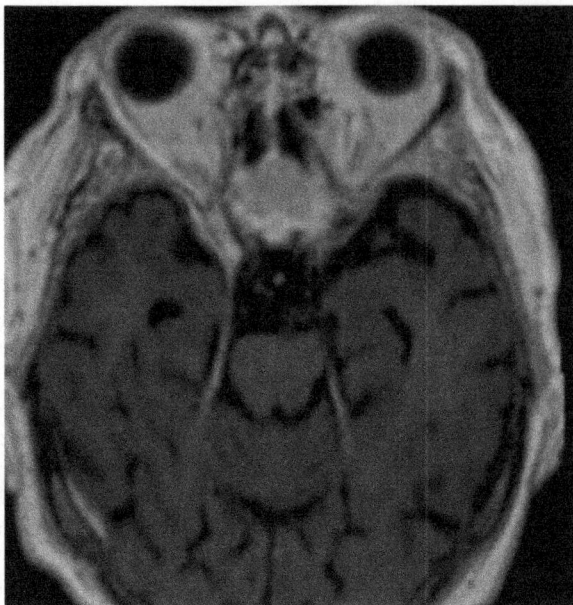

Figure 1.
MRI scan with gadolinium (Gd) of an olfactory groove meningioma.

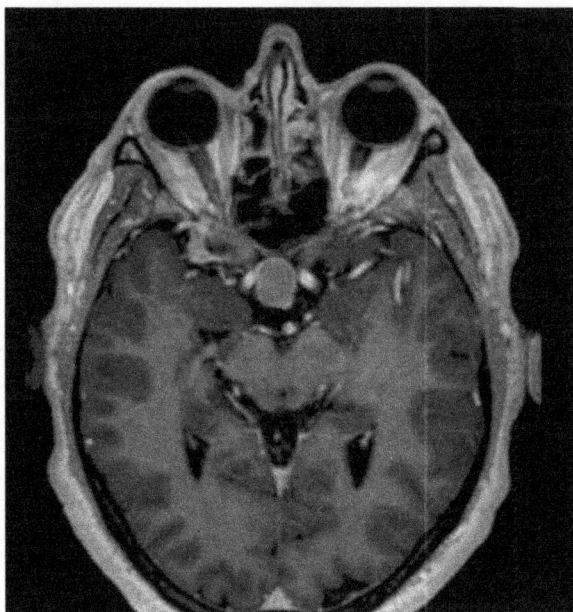

Figure 2.
MRI scan with Gd of a tuberculum sellae meningioma.

2.2 Pituitary adenomas

Pituitary adenomas are one of the most common intracranial tumors and are associated with a high rate of morbidity and mortality [25]. The prevalence of pituitary adenomas is approximately 100 per 100.000 [26–28]. Radical tumor resection is indicated, with a transsphenoidal approach [29]. Adenomas that secrete hormones are called functioning adenomas, and adenomas that do not secrete hormones are called nonfunctioning adenomas [28]. Nonfunctioning

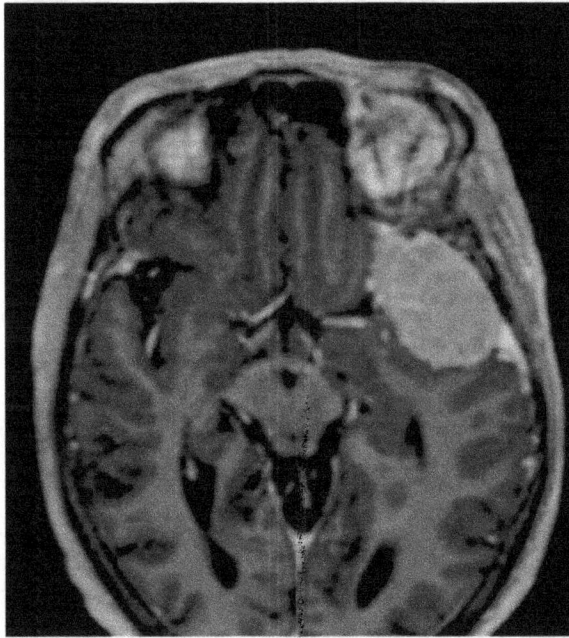

Figure 3.
MRI scan with Gd of a large left-sided sphenoid wing meningioma.

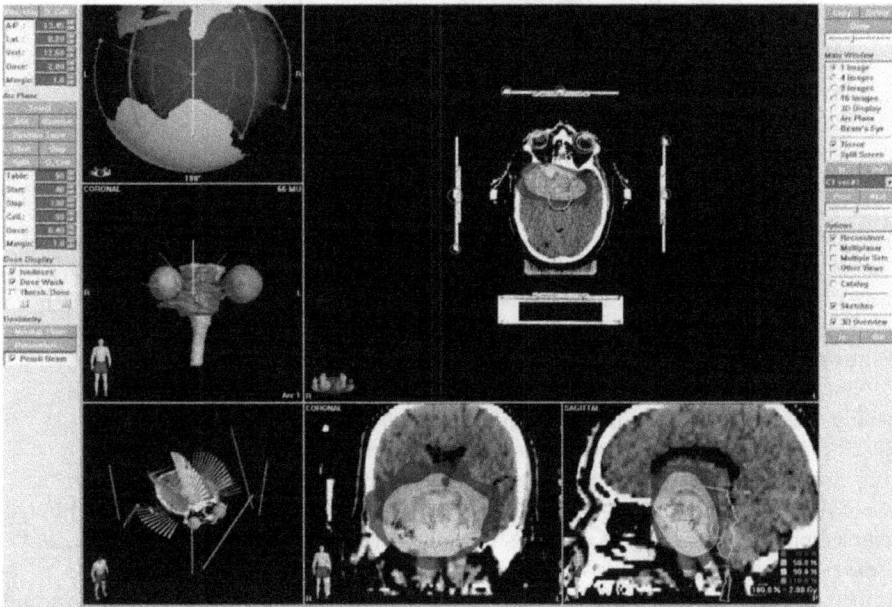

Figure 4.
Stereotactic radiation therapy dose plan in BrainLab/iPlan, of a right cavernous sinus meningioma, with isodose lines, demonstrating collateral irradiation of the optic chiasm, pituitary gland, and vascular structures of the cavernous sinus and circle of Willis.

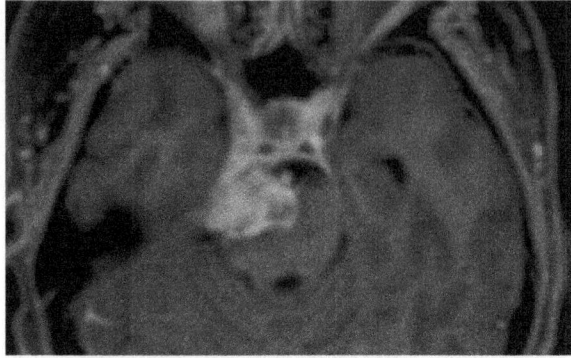

Figure 5.
MRI scan with Gd of a right petroclival meningioma.

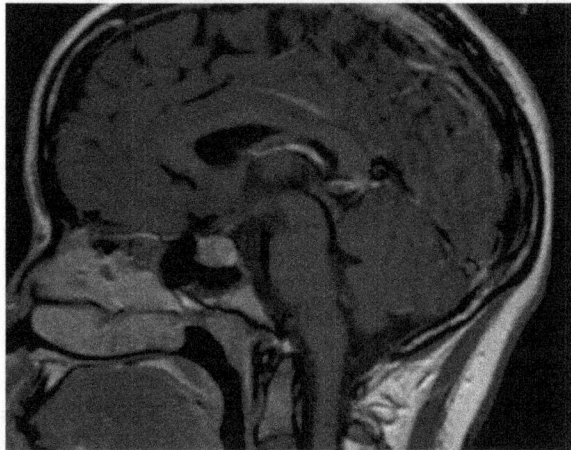

Figure 6.
MRI sagittal T1 with Gd of a pituitary microadenoma.

and prolactin-secreting adenomas are the most common types of pituitary adenomas, followed by growth hormone secreting and corticotroph adenomas, thyrotropin, and gonadotropin secretin) g adenomas [26, 28, 29]. Macroadenomas, which are defined as tumors with a diameter > 10 mm, are more common than microadenomas, which are <10 mm in diameter [28, 29]. The first-line treatment of prolactinomas is medical, with a dopamine agonist (**Figure 6**) [28].

Nonfunctioning pituitary adenomas are often large at presentation and are usually diagnosed due to their mass effect, visual loss, and hypopituitarism [27, 28]. Occasionally, they may constitute an asymptomatic incidental finding. They may also cause hyperprolactinemia due to pressure on the pituitary stalk. The main indication for surgery is reversal of visual loss, and in many cases, it may reverse hypopituitarism [29]. When surgical treatment does not provide sufficient disease control or has serious side effects, such as visual loss, then stereotactic radiosurgery or fractionated stereotactic radiation therapy is indicated, and in some instances, this may then be the sole treatment of the tumor (**Figure** 7). Also, stereotactic irradiation may be effective when surgery has failed to restore biochemical control in hormone-secreting adenomas [7].

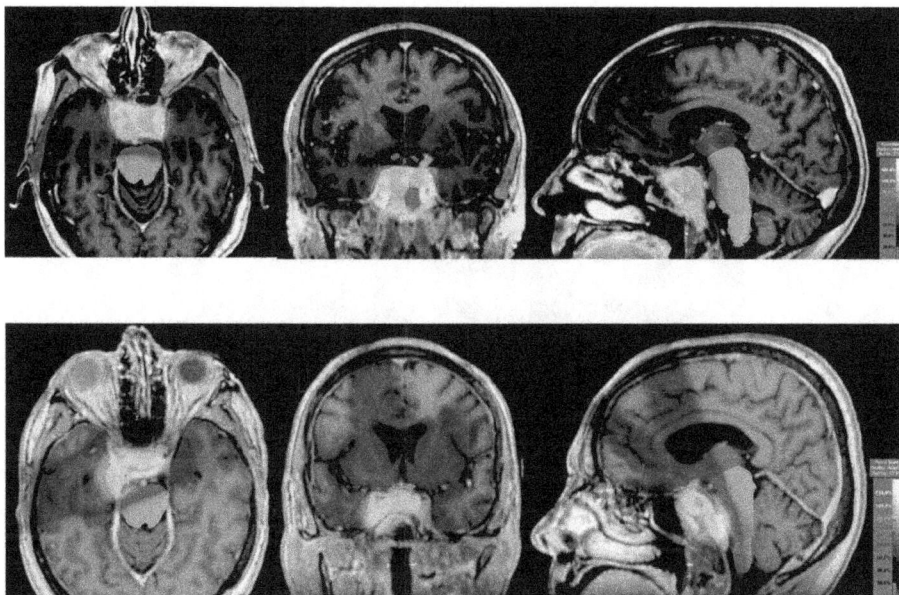

Figure 7.
FSRT dose plan of a large pituitary macroadenoma.

2.3 Craniopharyngiomas

Craniopharyngiomas are usually benign epithelial tumors originating from remnants of the Rathke's pouch, localized in the sellar or suprasellar region [30]. They are rare, with an incidence of 0.5–2 per 100,000 a year [31, 32]. They often present during childhood or adolescence and persist into adulthood [32]. They are cystic or solid or mixed cystic and solid and frequently contain calcifications (**Figure 8**) [31]. Presenting symptoms include visual field defects, pituitary hormone deficiency, and diabetes insipidus [30–32]. Craniopharyngiomas can be very challenging in terms of surgical management and can cause significant morbidity, despite their benign nature [33]. There are two distinct histological types of craniopharyngiomas. The adamantinomatous type is predominant in children, is more cystic and calcified and large, and often adherent to the brain. The less common papillary type almost exclusively presents in adults, is less infiltrative, and may be more amenable to surgery [34]. However, papillary craniopharyngiomas are well suited for stereotactic radiosurgery or fractionated stereotactic radiation therapy, as they are more radiosensitive and rarely recur after irradiation. Due to the high recurrence rate after subtotal resection, adjuvant irradiation is often warranted, with stereotactic radiosurgery or fractionated stereotactic radiation therapy [30, 35]. The main indication for stereotactic radiation therapy or stereotactic radiosurgery for craniopharyngiomas is thus when surgical control is not possible, or in case of tumor recurrence where the risks of surgery outweigh the benefits [36, 37].

2.4 Vestibular schwannomas

Vestibular schwannomas are slow-growing and benign tumors originating from the Schwann cell sheath of the cochleovestibular nerve (**Figure 9**) [38, 39]. The incidence is 1–2 in 100.000 a year [38, 39]. As the vestibular schwannomas grow, they affect hearing and balance, with unilateral hearing loss, tinnitus, and balance

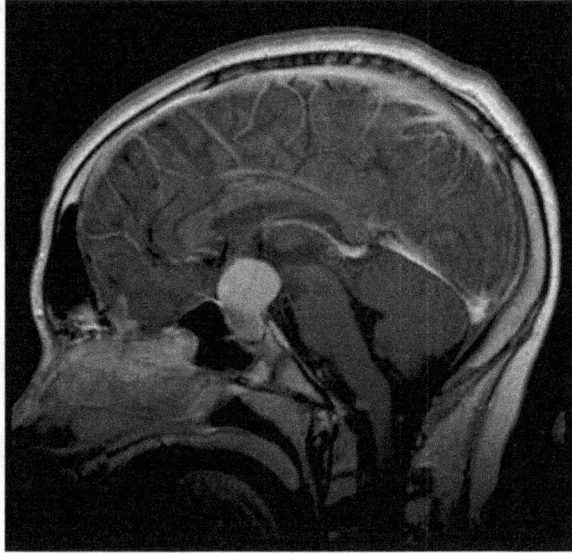

Figure 8.
MRI scan sagittal with Gd demonstrating a mainly solid craniopharyngioma in a 16-year-old adolescent.

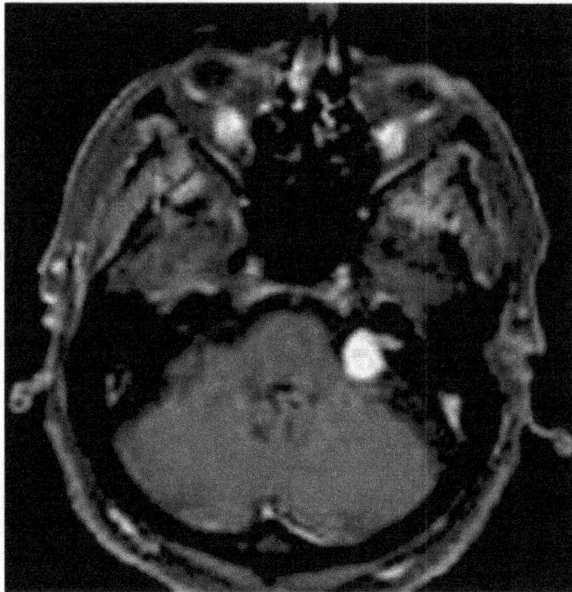

Figure 9.
MRI scan with Gd demonstrating a small left-sided vestibular schwannoma.

disturbances [39, 40]. With increasing tumor growth, the facial nerve can also be affected. Bilateral vestibular schwannomas with bilateral hearing loss are usually associated with neurofibromatosis type 2. Surgery is the standard treatment of vestibular schwannomas, including microsurgery and hearing preservation surgery [38]. More recently, stereotactic radiosurgery and radiation therapy have been introduced for the treatment of vestibular schwannomas with the aim of tumor control and hearing preservation, and controlled studies have found the results to be superior to microsurgery for small tumors less than 3 cm [38–40]. Sometimes a conservative wait and scan approach is appropriate, reserving treatment in case of tumor growth or neurological deterioration.

3. Tumor control and biochemical control

For skull base meningiomas, nonfunctioning pituitary adenomas, craniopharyngiomas, and vestibular schwannomas, the major goal of treatment is tumor control. Tumor control is defined as stable or reduced size of tumor after treatment. Long-term tumor control after fractionated stereotactic radiation therapy of benign anterior skull base tumors is well established from several large series and in several cases is superior to surgery, with long-term tumor control rates reported in the range of 88–100% for skull base meningiomas [4, 24, 41–46], 92–99% for pituitary adenomas [47–53], 75–100% for craniopharyngiomas [34, 37, 54, 55], and 85–100% for vestibular schwannomas [38, 40]. Long-term tumor control rates after stereotactic radiosurgery with LINAC or Gamma Knife have been reported to be similar [2, 4, 6, 8, 9, 36, 38, 56]. For hormone-secreting pituitary adenomas, an equally important goal of treatment is biochemical control [56]. For nonfunctioning pituitary adenomas, biochemical control rates of 50% of hormone-producing adenomas have been reported [7].

Tumor control can be evaluated on a contrast-enhanced MRI scan compared with the MRI scan before the radiation therapy. Pre- and post-therapy MRI and CT scans of the treatment plans are fused, with the gross tumor volume as reference [57]. Tumor volume is then calculated using 3D volumetric assessment with treatment planning software, i.e., from Electa, BrainLab, or Varian Eclipse. Tumor control is defined as stable size or regression of the tumor. A change in tumor volume by ≥25% can be considered a change in size, and a change in tumor volume < 25% can be considered stable size [34].

Serial neuroimaging follow-up until at least 10 years after treatment is generally recommended.

3.1 Visual complications

During the irradiation of tumors, with close anatomical relation to the optic chiasm and nerves, a certain degree of collateral irradiation of these intact but sensitive structures occurs [58, 59]. In therapy protocols, the optic nerves, chiasm, and tracts are usually outlined and defined as organs at risk (OAR) [57]. Radiation-induced optic neuropathy (RION) is defined as painless rapid visual loss and is attributed to radiation necrosis of the anterior optic pathways [60]. It often has a delayed onset and can result in either visual acuity or visual field loss. The risk of radiation-induced optic neuropathy is dependent on both the total cumulated radiation dose and the fraction dose [60]. The risk is markedly increased at cumulated optic chiasm radiation doses of ≥60 Gy in the case of fractionated stereotactic radiation therapy and at a single dose of >12 Gy in the case of radiosurgery [60]. The risk is greater with increasing age, preexisting compression of the optic nerves/chiasm, and previous radiation therapy. Percentages of 3–7 and 7–20% of RION in the dose ranges 55–60 and above 60 Gy, respectively, have been reported, as presented in the review by the QUANTEC initiative [60].

Fractionated stereotactic radiation therapy combines the advantage of a high accuracy of stereotactic technique and the biological advantage of fractionation [1, 48]. For stereotactic radiosurgery (SRS) of tumors in the vicinity of the optic structures, there is a dose-limiting factor, meaning that the minimal effective tumor dose may be equal to or greater than the dose tolerated by the optic structures. For example, the treatment of tumors of the cavernous sinus, with single-dose SRS, has been shown not to affect the optic pathways at a single dose of <10, whereas the incidence of optic neuropathy has been shown to be 27% after a single dose of 10 Gy–15 Gy and 78% after a single dose of >15 Gy [58]. Other SRS studies of perioptic tumors have reported variable results [4–6, 61–64].

3.2 Hypopituitarism

The pituitary gland is particularly sensitive to radiation, and hypopituitarism is the most common side effect after radiation therapy [65]. When high-dose radiation is applied directly to the pituitary gland for the treatment of pituitary adenomas, frequently it results in pituitary deficiency of one or more hormonal axes, and this correlates well with radiation dose to the pituitary gland [65, 66]. Furthermore, radiation damage of the hypothalamus can result in hypopituitarism [50]. Treatment requiring hypopituitarism of one or more hormonal axes has been reported in around 8% of these patients [7].

3.3 Cerebral infarction

Occlusion of the carotid artery or its branches leading to cerebral infarction or ischemic stroke is a potentially serious and life-threatening complication after stereotactic radiation therapy involving the extra- or intracavernous portion of the carotid artery or the Circle of Willis [67]. Although considered to be relatively rare, radiation-induced cerebral infarction has been reported after single fraction stereotactic radiosurgery or radiation therapy of meningiomas, pituitary adenomas, craniopharyngiomas, and vestibular schwannomas, with an occurrence of 1–7% [24, 46, 68–70]. However, the risk of cerebral infarction may not be increased when compared with the incidence in the general population. Predisposing risk factors identified for ischemic events are smoking, hypertension, and hyperlipidemia, as well as increased age [70]. Cerebral infarction is by definition a clinical diagnosis; therefore, subclinical infarctions only detectable by neuroimaging may occur [70].

3.4 Hearing loss

Both stereotactic radiosurgery and fractionated stereotactic radiation therapy have been shown to accelerate the naturally occurring hearing loss in patients in around 50% of treated patients with vestibular schwannoma, and the degree of hearing loss is correlated to the radiation dose to the cochlea [38, 40].

3.5 Malignancies

The occurrence of intracranial malignancies after conventional radiation therapy is well known but is not well established following stereotactic radiation therapy and radiosurgery, but since this is often a late event, existing studies may not have had long enough follow-up. It would be feasible to conduct such a study, but with very long-term (10–20 years) follow-up.

4. Conclusions

Benign anterior skull base tumors include meningiomas, pituitary adenomas, craniopharyngiomas, and vestibular schwannomas. As an adjuvant therapy to surgery or when surgical treatment carries too high a risk of complications, a highly precise focused radiation, known as fractionated stereotactic radiation therapy (FSRT) or stereotactic radiosurgery (SRS) can be delivered to the tumor. Treatment modalities include Gamma Knife for SRS, LINAC for FSRT/SRS, Cyberknife for SRS or hypo fractionated FSRT, and more recently, proton beam therapy. FSRT in particular combines the high accuracy of stereotactic radiosurgery and the benefit of fractionation. Existing studies include systematic analysis of complications and risk factors FSRT/SRS of tumors with localizations relating to vision, hormone-secreting regions, cerebral vasculature, and hearing. Paying attention to risk reduction is extremely important to prevent complications. Existing studies provide evidence of good long-term tumor control for benign tumors of the skull base. Upweighting the risks against surgical complications and uncontrolled tumor growth, stereotactic radiotherapy and radiosurgery appear to be relatively safe as a treatment of patients with benign anterior skull base tumors. However, improved dose planning techniques may be able to reduce the incidence of side effects further. Further studies with very long-time follow-up including the potential for malignancy are needed.

Conflict of interest

The author declares no conflict of interest.

Thanks

Special thanks to Tina Obbekjaer, Mahmoud Albarazi, and Marianne Juhler, for their advice during the preparation of this book chapter.

Author details

Arnar Astradsson
Department of Neurosurgery, Aarhus University Hospital, Aarhus N, Denmark

*Address all correspondence to: arnar.astradsson@gmail.com

IntechOpen

References

[1] Friedman WA, Buatti JM, Bova FJ, Mendenhall WL. Linac Radiosurgery A Practical Guide. New York: Springer; 1998. p. 176

[2] Lindquist C. Gamma knife surgery: Evolution and long-term results. In: Kondziolka D, editor. Radiosurgery. Basel: Karger; 1999. pp. 1-12

[3] Kondziolka D, Shin SM, Brunswick A, Kim I, Silverman JS. The biology of radiosurgery and its clinical applications for brain tumors. Neuro-Oncology. 2015;**17**(1):29-44

[4] Spiegelmann R, Cohen ZR, Nissim O, Alezra D, Pfeffer R. Cavernous sinus meningiomas: A large LINAC radiosurgery series. Journal of Neuro-Oncology. 2010;**98**(2):195-202

[5] Spiegelmann R, Nissim O, Menhel J, Alezra D, Pfeffer MR. Linear accelerator radiosurgery for meningiomas in and around the cavernous sinus. Neurosurgery. 2002;**51**(6):1373-1379

[6] Runge MJ, Maarouf M, Hunsche S, Kocher M, Ruge MI, El Majdoub F, et al. LINAC-radiosurgery for nonsecreting pituitary adenomas. Long-term results. Strahlentherapie und Onkologie. 2012;**188**(4):319-325

[7] Roug S, Rasmussen AK, Juhler M, Kosteljanetz M, Poulsgaard L, Heeboll H, et al. Fractionated stereotactic radiotherapy in patients with acromegaly: An interim single-centre audit. European Journal of Endocrinology. 2010;**162**(4):685-694

[8] Mirza B, Monsted A, Harding J, Ohlhues L, Roed H, Juhler M. Stereotactic radiotherapy and radiosurgery in pediatric patients: Analysis of indications and outcome. Child's Nervous System. 2010;**26**(12):1785-1793

[9] Pollock BE, Cochran J, Natt N, Brown PD, Erickson D, Link MJ, et al. Gamma knife radiosurgery for patients with nonfunctioning pituitary adenomas: Results from a 15-year experience. International Journal of Radiation Oncology, Biology, Physics. 2008;**70**(5):1325-1329

[10] Adler JR Jr, Gibbs IC, Puataweepong P, Chang SD. Visual field preservation after multisession cyberknife radiosurgery for perioptic lesions. Neurosurgery. 2008;**62**(Suppl. 2):733-743

[11] Ahmed KA, Demetriou SK, McDonald M, Johnstone PA. Clinical benefits of proton beam therapy for tumors of the skull base. Cancer Control. 2016;**23**(3):213-219

[12] Bishop AJ, Greenfield B, Mahajan A, Paulino AC, Okcu MF, Allen PK, et al. Proton beam therapy versus conformal photon radiation therapy for childhood craniopharyngioma: Multi-institutional analysis of outcomes, cyst dynamics, and toxicity. International Journal of Radiation Oncology, Biology, Physics. 2014;**90**(2):354-361

[13] Rockhill J, Mrugala M, Chamberlain MC. Intracranial meningiomas: An overview of diagnosis and treatment. Neurosurgical Focus. 2007;**23**(4):E1

[14] Wiemels J, Wrensch M, Claus EB. Epidemiology and etiology of meningioma. Journal of Neuro-Oncology. 2010;**99**(3):307-314

[15] Louis DN, Ohgaki H, Wiestler OD, Cavenee WK, Burger PC, Jouvet A, et al. The 2007 WHO classification of tumours of the central nervous system. Acta Neuropathologica. 2007;**114**(2): 97-109

[16] Kleihues P, Burger PC, Scheithauer BW. The new WHO

classification of brain tumours. Brain Pathology. 1993;**3**(3):255-268

[17] Kleihues P, Louis DN, Scheithauer BW, Rorke LB, Reifenberger G, Burger PC, et al. The WHO classification of tumors of the nervous system. Journal of Neuropathology and Experimental Neurology. 2002;**61**(3):215-225

[18] Simpson D. The recurrence of intracranial meningiomas after surgical treatment. Journal of Neurology, Neurosurgery, and Psychiatry. 1957;**20**(1):22-39

[19] Rachinger W, Grau S, Tonn JC. Different microsurgical approaches to meningiomas of the anterior cranial base. Acta Neurochirurgica. 2010;**152**(6):931-939

[20] Hentschel SJ, DeMonte F. Olfactory groove meningiomas. Neurosurgical Focus. 2003;**14**(6):e4

[21] Erkmen K, Pravdenkova S, Al-Mefty O. Surgical management of petroclival meningiomas: Factors determining the choice of approach. Neurosurgical Focus. 2005;**19**(2):E7

[22] Heth JA, Al-Mefty O. Cavernous sinus meningiomas. Neurosurgical Focus. 2003;**14**(6):e3

[23] Brell M, Villa S, Teixidor P, Lucas A, Ferran E, Marin S, et al. Fractionated stereotactic radiotherapy in the treatment of exclusive cavernous sinus meningioma: Functional outcome, local control, and tolerance. Surgical Neurology. 2006;**65**(1):28-33

[24] Pollock BE, Stafford SL, Link MJ, Garces YI, Foote RL. Single-fraction radiosurgery of benign cavernous sinus meningiomas. Journal of Neurosurgery. 2013;**119**(3):675-682

[25] Castinetti F, Regis J, Dufour H, Brue T. Role of stereotactic radiosurgery in the management of pituitary adenomas. Nature Reviews. Endocrinology. 2010;**6**(4):214-223

[26] Fernandez A, Karavitaki N, Wass JA. Prevalence of pituitary adenomas: A community-based, cross-sectional study in Banbury (Oxfordshire, UK). Clinical Endocrinology. 2010;**72**(3):377-382

[27] Chanson P, Raverot G, Castinetti F, Cortet-Rudelli C, Galland F, Salenave S, et al. Management of clinically non-functioning pituitary adenoma. Annales d'endocrinologie. 2015;**76**(3):239-247

[28] Rogers A, Karavitaki N, Wass JA. Diagnosis and management of prolactinomas and non-functioning pituitary adenomas. BMJ. 2014;**349**:g5390

[29] Berkmann S, Fandino J, Muller B, Kothbauer KF, Henzen C, Landolt H. Pituitary surgery: Experience from a large network in Central Switzerland. Swiss Medical Weekly. 2012;**142**:w13680

[30] Karavitaki N, Cudlip S, Adams CB, Wass JA. Craniopharyngiomas. Endocrine Reviews. 2006;**27**(4):371-397

[31] Erfurth EM, Holmer H, Fjalldal SB. Mortality and morbidity in adult craniopharyngioma. Pituitary. 2013;**16**(1):46-55

[32] Trippel M, Nikkhah G. Stereotactic neurosurgical treatment options for craniopharyngioma. Frontiers in Endocrinology (Lausanne). 2012;**3**:63

[33] Fahlbusch R, Honegger J, Paulus W, Huk W, Buchfelder M. Surgical treatment of craniopharyngiomas: Experience with 168 patients. Journal of Neurosurgery. 1999;**90**(2):237-250

[34] Astradsson A, Munck Af Rosenschöld P, Feldt-Rasmussen U, Poulsgaard L, Wiencke AK, Ohlhues L, et al. Visual outcome, endocrine

function and tumor control after fractionated stereotactic radiation therapy of craniopharyngiomas in adults: Findings in a prospective cohort. Acta Oncologica. Mar 2017;**56**(3): 415-421

[35] Ulfarsson E, Lindquist C, Roberts M, Rahn T, Lindquist M, Thoren M, et al. Gamma knife radiosurgery for craniopharyngiomas: Long-term results in the first Swedish patients. Journal of Neurosurgery. 2002;**97**(Suppl. 5):613-622

[36] Chung WY, Pan DH, Shiau CY, Guo WY, Wang LW. Gamma knife radiosurgery for craniopharyngiomas. Journal of Neurosurgery. 2000;**93** (Suppl. 3):47-56

[37] Combs SE, Thilmann C, Huber PE, Hoess A, Debus J, Schulz-Ertner D. Achievement of long-term local control in patients with craniopharyngiomas using high precision stereotactic radiotherapy. Cancer. 2007;**109**(11):2308-2314

[38] Persson O, Jr B, Shalom NB, Wangerid T, Jakola AS, Förander P. Stereotactic radiosurgery vs. fractionated radiotherapy for tumor control in vestibular schwannoma patients: A systematic review. Acta Neurochirurgica. 2017;**159**(6):1013-1021

[39] Baschnagel AM, Chen PY, Bojrab D, Pieper D, Kartush J, Didyuk O, et al. Hearing preservation in patients with vestibular schwannoma treated with Gamma Knife surgery. Journal of Neurosurgery. 2013;**118**(3):571-578

[40] Rasmussen R, Claesson M, Stangerup SE, Roed H, Christensen IJ, Caye-Thomasen P, et al. Fractionated stereotactic radiotherapy of vestibular schwannomas accelerates hearing loss. International Journal of Radiation Oncology, Biology, Physics. 2012;**83**(5):e607-e611

[41] Stiebel-Kalish H, Reich E, Gal L, Rappaport ZH, Nissim O, Pfeffer R, et al. Visual outcome in meningiomas around anterior visual pathways treated with linear accelerator fractionated stereotactic radiotherapy. International Journal of Radiation Oncology, Biology, Physics. 2012;**82**(2):779-788

[42] Metellus P, Batra S, Karkar S, Kapoor S, Weiss S, Kleinberg L, et al. Fractionated conformal radiotherapy in the management of cavernous sinus meningiomas: Long-term functional outcome and tumor control at a single institution. International Journal of Radiation Oncology, Biology, Physics. 2010;**78**(3):836-843

[43] Hamm K, Henzel M, Gross MW, Surber G, Kleinert G, Engenhart-Cabillic R. Radiosurgery/ stereotactic radiotherapy in the therapeutical concept for skull base meningiomas. Zentralblatt für Neurochirurgie. 2008;**69**(1):14-21

[44] Henzel M, Gross MW, Hamm K, Surber G, Kleinert G, Failing T, et al. Stereotactic radiotherapy of meningiomas: Symptomatology, acute and late toxicity. Strahlentherapie und Onkologie. 2006;**182**(7):382-388

[45] Jalali R, Loughrey C, Baumert B, Perks J, Warrington AP, Traish D, et al. High precision focused irradiation in the form of fractionated stereotactic conformal radiotherapy (SCRT) for benign meningiomas predominantly in the skull base location. Clinical Oncology (Royal College of Radiologists). 2002;**14**(2):103-109

[46] Pollock BE, Stafford SL. Results of stereotactic radiosurgery for patients with imaging defined cavernous sinus meningiomas. International Journal of Radiation Oncology, Biology, Physics. 2005;**62**(5):1427-1431

[47] Minniti G, Traish D, Ashley S, Gonsalves A, Brada M. Fractionated

stereotactic conformal radiotherapy for secreting and nonsecreting pituitary adenomas. Clinical Endocrinology. 2006;**64**(5):542-548

[48] Elhateer H, Muanza T, Roberge D, Ruo R, Eldebawy E, Lambert C, et al. Fractionated stereotactic radiotherapy in the treatment of pituitary macroadenomas. Current Oncology. 2008;**15**(6):286-292

[49] Milker-Zabel S, Debus J, Thilmann C, Schlegel W, Wannenmacher M. Fractionated stereotactically guided radiotherapy and radiosurgery in the treatment of functional and nonfunctional adenomas of the pituitary gland. International Journal of Radiation Oncology, Biology, Physics. 2001;**50**(5):1279-1286

[50] Paek SH, Downes MB, Bednarz G, Keane WM, Werner-Wasik M, Curran WJ Jr, et al. Integration of surgery with fractionated stereotactic radiotherapy for treatment of nonfunctioning pituitary macroadenomas. International Journal of Radiation Oncology, Biology, Physics. 2005;**61**(3):795-808

[51] Colin P, Jovenin N, Delemer B, Caron J, Grulet H, Hecart AC, et al. Treatment of pituitary adenomas by fractionated stereotactic radiotherapy: A prospective study of 110 patients. International Journal of Radiation Oncology, Biology, Physics. 2005;**62**(2):333-341

[52] Kopp C, Theodorou M, Poullos N, Jacob V, Astner ST, Molls M, et al. Tumor shrinkage assessed by volumetric MRI in long-term follow-up after fractionated stereotactic radiotherapy of nonfunctioning pituitary adenoma. International Journal of Radiation Oncology, Biology, Physics. 2012;**82**(3):1262-1267

[53] Weber DC, Momjian S, Pralong FP, Meyer P, Villemure JG, Pica A. Adjuvant

or radical fractionated stereotactic radiotherapy for patients with pituitary functional and nonfunctional macroadenoma. Radiation Oncology. 2011;**6**:169

[54] Harrabi SB, Adeberg S, Welzel T, Rieken S, Habermehl D, Debus J, et al. Long term results after fractionated stereotactic radiotherapy (FSRT) in patients with craniopharyngioma: Maximal tumor control with minimal side effects. Radiation Oncology. 2014;**9**:203

[55] Minniti G, Saran F, Traish D, Soomal R, Sardell S, Gonsalves A, et al. Fractionated stereotactic conformal radiotherapy following conservative surgery in the control of craniopharyngiomas. Radiotherapy and Oncology. 2007;**82**(1):90-95

[56] Pollock BE, Nippoldt TB, Stafford SL, Foote RL, Abboud CF. Results of stereotactic radiosurgery in patients with hormone-producing pituitary adenomas: Factors associated with endocrine normalization. Journal of Neurosurgery. 2002;**97**(3):525-530

[57] Astradsson A, Wiencke AK, Munck af Rosenschold P, Engelholm SA, Ohlhues L, Roed H, et al. Visual outcome after fractionated stereotactic radiation therapy of benign anterior skull base tumors. Journal of Neuro-Oncology. 2014;**118**(1):101-108

[58] Leber KA, Bergloff J, Pendl G. Dose-response tolerance of the visual pathways and cranial nerves of the cavernous sinus to stereotactic radiosurgery. Journal of Neurosurgery. 1998;**88**(1):43-50

[59] Nutting C, Brada M, Brazil L, Sibtain A, Saran F, Westbury C, et al. Radiotherapy in the treatment of benign meningioma of the skull base. Journal of Neurosurgery. 1999;**90**(5):823-827

[60] Mayo C, Martel MK, Marks LB, Flickinger J, Nam J, Kirkpatrick J.

Radiation dose-volume effects of optic nerves and chiasm. International Journal of Radiation Oncology, Biology, Physics. 2010;**76**(Suppl. 3):S28-S35

[61] Morita A, Coffey RJ, Foote RL, Schiff D, Gorman D. Risk of injury to cranial nerves after gamma knife radiosurgery for skull base meningiomas: Experience in 88 patients. Journal of Neurosurgery. 1999;**90**(1):42-49

[62] Stafford SL, Pollock BE, Leavitt JA, Foote RL, Brown PD, Link MJ, et al. A study on the radiation tolerance of the optic nerves and chiasm after stereotactic radiosurgery. International Journal of Radiation Oncology, Biology, Physics. 2003;**55**(5):1177-1181

[63] Cifarelli CP, Schlesinger DJ, Sheehan JP. Cranial nerve dysfunction following Gamma Knife surgery for pituitary adenomas: Long-term incidence and risk factors. Journal of Neurosurgery. 2012;**116**(6):1304-1310

[64] Tishler RB, Loeffler JS, Lunsford LD, Duma C, Alexander E 3rd, Kooy HM, et al. Tolerance of cranial nerves of the cavernous sinus to radiosurgery. International Journal of Radiation Oncology, Biology, Physics. 1993;**27**(2):215-221

[65] Littley MD, Shalet SM, Beardwell CG, Ahmed SR, Applegate G, Sutton ML. Hypopituitarism following external radiotherapy for pituitary tumours in adults. The Quarterly Journal of Medicine. 1989;**70**(262):145-160

[66] Littley MD, Shalet SM, Beardwell CG, Robinson EL, Sutton ML. Radiation-induced hypopituitarism is dose-dependent. Clinical Endocrinology. 1989;**31**(3):363-373

[67] Scoccianti S, Detti B, Gadda D, Greto D, Furfaro I, Meacci F, et al. Organs at risk in the brain and their dose-constraints in adults and in children: A radiation oncologist's guide for delineation in everyday practice. Radiotherapy and Oncology. 2015;**114**(2):230-238

[68] Correa SF, Marta GN, Teixeira MJ. Neurosymptomatic carvenous sinus meningioma: A 15-years experience with fractionated stereotactic radiotherapy and radiosurgery. Radiation Oncology. 2014;**9**:27

[69] Lim YJ, Leem W, Park JT, Kim TS, Rhee BA, Kim GK. Cerebral infarction with ICA occlusion after Gamma Knife radiosurgery for pituitary adenoma: A case report. Stereotactic and Functional Neurosurgery. 1999;**72**(Suppl. 1):132-139

[70] Astradsson A, Munck Af Rosenschöld P, Poulsgaard L, Ohlhues L, Engelholm SA, Feldt-Rasmussen U, et al. Cerebral infarction after fractionated stereotactic radiation therapy of benign anterior skull base tumors. Clinical and Translational Radiation Oncology. 2019;**7**(15):93-98

Section 3

Meningiomas of the Skull Base

Chapter 3

Spheno-Orbital Meningiomas

Guillaume Baucher, Lucas Troude and Pierre-Hugues Roche

Abstract

Spheno-orbital meningiomas are mainly defined as primary *en plaque* tumors of the lesser and greater sphenoid wings, invading the underlying bone and adjacent anatomical structures. The patients, mostly women in their fifties, generally present with a progressive, unilateral, and nonpulsatile proptosis, often associated with cosmetic deformity and optic nerve damage. Surgical resection is currently the gold standard of treatment in case of optic neuropathy, significant symptoms, or radiological progression. The surgical strategy should take into account the morphology of the tumor, its epicenter at the level of the sphenoid wing, and the invasion of adjacent anatomical structures. Surgery stabilizes or improves visual function and oculomotricity in most cases but it is rare that the proptosis recovers completely. Gross total resection is hard to achieve considering the complex anatomy of the spheno-orbital region and the risk of inducing cranial nerve deficits. Rare cases of WHO grade II or III meningiomas warrant adjuvant radiotherapy. Tumor residues after subtotal resections of WHO grade I meningiomas are first radiologically monitored and then treated by stereotactic radiosurgery in case of progression.

Keywords: meningioma, spheno-orbital meningioma, optic nerve, optic canal, anterior clinoid process, superior orbital fissure, sphenoid wing, cavernous sinus, proptosis

1. Introduction

As early as 1922, Harvey Cushing distinguished two types of meningiomas: spherical *en masse* tumors with lobulated and sometimes irregular growth, and *en plaque* tumors, which are slightly elevated from and extend along the inner dural layer [1, 2]. *En plaque* meningiomas are classically associated with significant underlying hyperostosis caused by tumor invasion of the bone and overexpression of osteogenic molecules influencing the osteoblast/osteoclast activity (e.g., osteoprotegerin and insulin-like growth factor 1), [3, 4]. Their preferred location in the pterional region and the sphenoid ridge could be due to the important intraosseous branching of meningeal vessels and venous sinuses at this level [1, 5]. Due to the anatomical complexity of this region, many different names have been used to describe this pathological entity (e.g., *en plaque* sphenoid wing meningioma, *en plaque* pterional meningioma, invading meningioma of the sphenoid ridge, hyperostoting meningioma of the sphenoid ridge, pterional-orbital meningioma...); however, spheno-orbital meningioma (SOM) seems to be both the most appropriate and the most frequently used term [6]. Consequently, SOMs are mainly defined as primary *en plaque* tumors of the lesser and greater sphenoid wings that invade the underlying bone and potentially adjacent anatomical structures [7]. They can progressively extend to the temporal and infratemporal fossae, orbit, anterior clinoid process

(ACP) and cavernous sinus (CS), compromising the integrity of the optic canal, the superior orbital fissure (SOF), and the cranial nerves passing through [8].

2. Epidemiological data and clinical presentation

While meningiomas account for approximately 20% of all intracranial tumors in males and 38% in females (with a 2:1 female-to-male ratio) [9, 10], SOMs comprise between 4% and 9% of all meningiomas [11]. In a meta-analysis of 38 retrospective studies about SOM that included a total of 1486 patients, Fisher *et al.* reported a mean age of 51 ± 6 years old, with a high proportion of women (82%) [12].

In a review of the literature, Apra *et al.* demonstrated a greater female predominance in SOM (86% across 14 different series with a total of 867 patients) than in meningiomas from all locations (74% female in a total of 110,359 patients in the largest meningioma study) [13, 14]. In their own retrospective study of 175 histologically confirmed cases of SOM, women were found to be significantly younger than men at the time of diagnosis (51 ± 5 vs. 63 ± 8 years) [13]. Notably, progesterone receptors were identified much more frequently in women than in men (96% vs. 50%), and exogenous hormone intake (predominantly progesterone) was identified in 83% of women in this same series, indicating that this is a risk factor for developing SOM [13].

Patients typically present with progressive, unilateral, and nonpulsatile proptosis (84%), often associated with cosmetic deformity [12, 15]. The frequent optic nerve (ON) disturbances result in unilateral decreased visual acuity (46%), constricted visual field (31%), and sometimes loss of color vision (5%) [12]. Ophthalmoplegia is seen in 25% of patients with SOM, often due to cranial oculomotor nerves deficit (oculomotor nerve 11%; trochlear nerve 6%; abducens nerve 4%). Diplopia can also be caused by intraorbital compression of the oculomotor muscles. Deficits in other cranial nerves (trigeminal, vestibulocochlear, and facial nerves) are less common. Finally, other general neurological signs, such as headaches (25%) and epileptic seizures (4%), are observed in patients with SOM.

3. Preoperative assessment

Skull radiographs were historically used to diagnose SOM by demonstrating unilateral sphenoid hyperostosis. With the emergence of computed tomography (CT) and magnetic resonance imaging (MRI), these techniques became the standard before any surgical procedure involving the removal of a SOM.

CT precisely demonstrates the bone features of the SOM, as well as its extension (**Figures 1** and **2**). Using CT, the involvement of the orbit walls, floor of the middle cranial fossa (including the foramens rotundum and ovale), SOF, ACP, and optic canal can be easily identified.

MRI completes the radiological assessment, showing the globoid or plaque-like shape of the intradural portion of the meningioma and its impact on the brain parenchyma (mass effect and edema). The epicenter of the tumor on the sphenoid wing is identified, and the specific involvement of the temporal and infratemporal fossae, orbit, SOF, optic canal, and CS is determined. At this stage, it is important to differentiate between simple involvement of the lateral wall of the CS and true intracompartment invasion. Similarly, the presence of meningioma within the optic canal or SOF should be similarly distinguished from tumor bony involvement of these structures (**Figures 1** and **2**). All of these details are critical, as they contribute to the planning of the upcoming surgical procedure for optimal tumor resection.

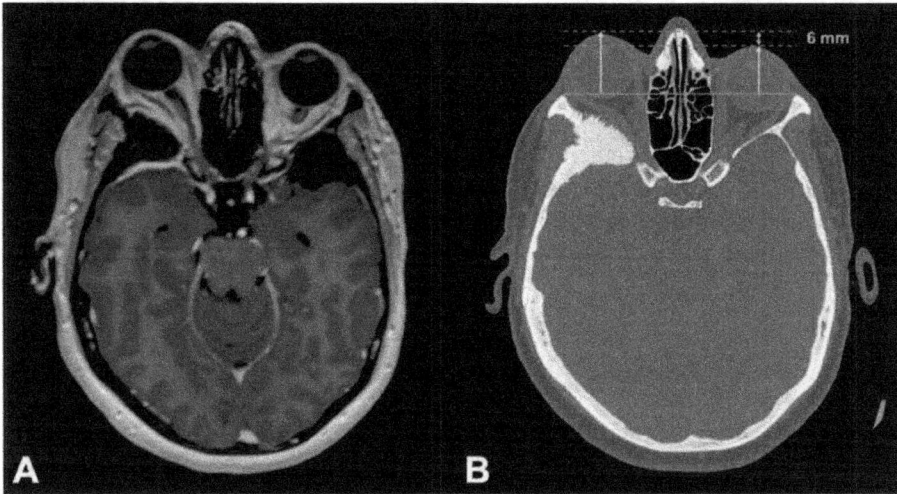

Figure 1.
(a) Axial contrast-enhanced T1-weighted magnetic resonance imaging demonstrates thickening of the temporopolar dura mater on the right side, with a deviated optic nerve compared to the left side. A temporopolar arachnoid cyst is seen on the left side. (b) Axial computed tomographic scan shows hyperostosis of both the lesser and greater sphenoid wings, sparing the anterior clinoid process. Proptosis can be easily measured on axial brain slices passing through the lens on both sides, by firstly taking as reference the line joining the two lateral orbital margins. This line is then projected to the level of each cornea and the distance between these two new lines is measured, giving an accurate and relevant estimate of proptosis for follow-up.

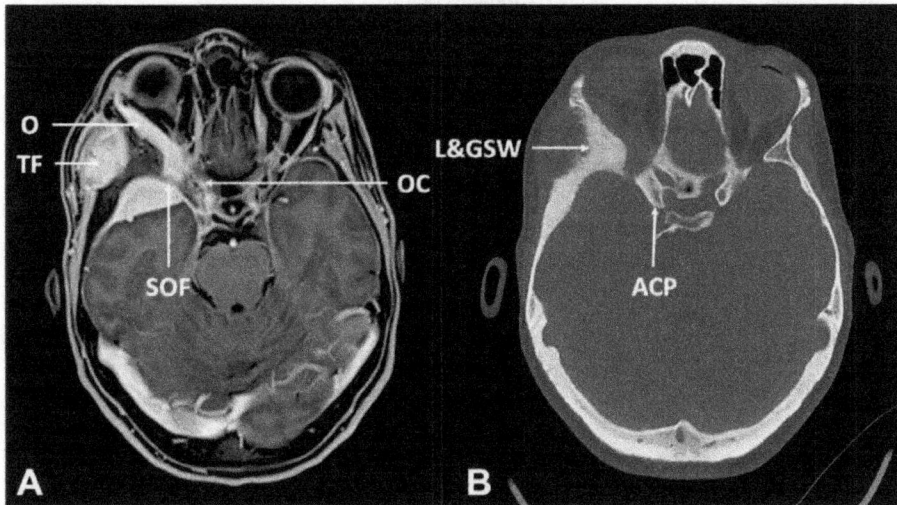

Figure 2.
(a) Axial contrast-enhanced T1-weighted magnetic resonance imaging demonstrates a large right spheno-orbital meningioma with middle sphenoid wing center, invading the temporal fossa (TF), the superior orbital fissure (SOF), and the orbit (O). There was no true invasion of the optic canal (OC) by the meningioma on thin-section MRI analysis. (b) Axial computed tomographic scan shows hyperostosis of the lesser and greater sphenoid wings (L&GSW) and anterior clinoid process (ACP) on the right side.

A comprehensive preoperative ophthalmological exam is mandatory and should include at least an objective assessment of visual acuity and field, a dilated-pupil fundus examination and ideally an optical coherence tomography (OCT). The Lancaster red-green test for assessment of oculomotor muscle function is performed according to the presence of diplopia. Accurate measurement of the proptosis can be achieved with an exophthalmometer or with correctly oriented cerebral imaging (**Figure 1**).

4. Differential diagnosis

At this time, differential diagnosis for hyperostosis due to SOM should also be considered. These include fibrous dysplasia, osteoma, osteoblastoma, Paget's disease, hyperostosis frontalis interna, osteoblastic metastases, and erythroid hyperplasia [15].

5. Therapeutic strategy and decision-making algorithm

As with all other meningiomas, the decision-making process for SOM must be tailored to each patient. Mass effect of the tumor, age, general condition, comorbidities, symptomatology, its impact on daily life, and the patient's wishes must be taken into account. In cases with absent or mild symptoms without mass effect on imaging, simple clinical and radiological monitoring can be chosen initially, with patient follow-up on a regular basis (every 3–6 months). In contrast, the presence of optic neuropathy, severe neurological symptoms, significant proptosis, or serious mass effect warrants surgical operation. Although a subject of debate, optimal

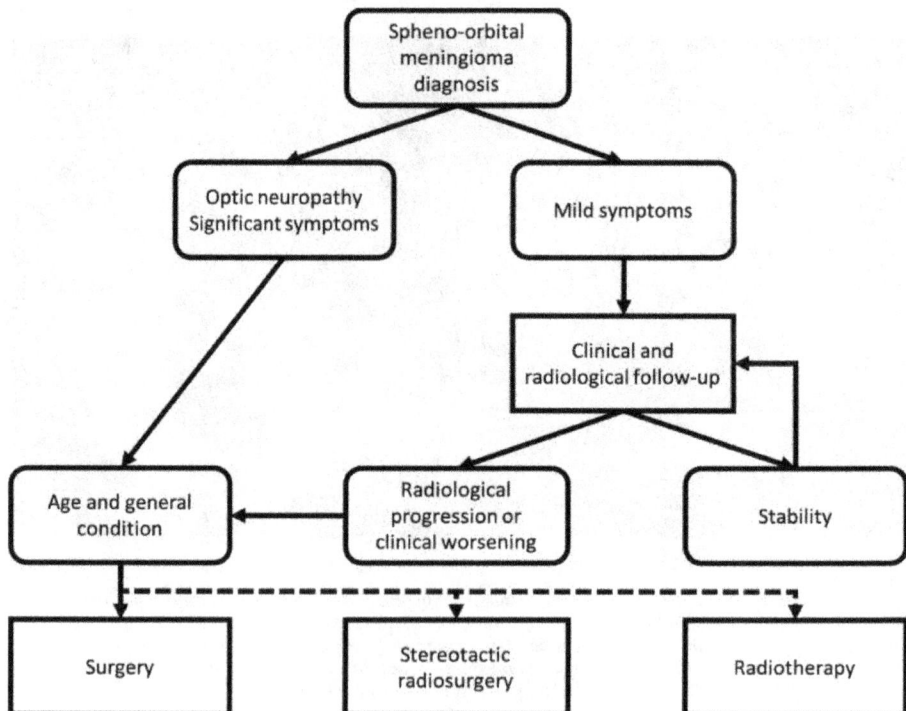

Figure 3.
Decision-making algorithm of first-line treatment for spheno-orbitary meningiomas, in accordance with the 2016 EANO guidelines [16]. The choice of radiation treatment is mainly based on the tumor volume, stereotactic radiosurgery being preferred for smaller tumors and radiotherapy being preferred for larger tumors.

surgical resection remains the current reference treatment for SOM, in accordance with the general EANO (European Association of Neuro-Oncology) guidelines for the management of meningiomas published in 2016 [16]. If the patient is in a fragile state of health or categorically refuses the operation, radiation treatment may be offered as an alternative. The choice of technique is then mainly based on the tumor volume, stereotactic radiosurgery being preferred for smaller tumors and radiotherapy being preferred for larger tumors. To summarize this reasoning, we propose a simple algorithm highlighting the main points to be taken into account during decision-making in cases of SOM (**Figure 3**).

6. Classification

Despite their common features, SOMs are a heterogeneous group of tumors due to the complex anatomy of the sphenoid bone, which is a part of both the skull base and the orbit. Few attempts have been made to classify SOMs. Roser *et al.* approached the classification of SOMs by first identifying the morphology of the meningioma (globoid, *en plaque,* and purely intraosseous), then detailing the involvement of the sphenoid wing and the CS [17]. Kong *et al.* in turn proposed a slightly simplified version, focusing on the location of the tumor epicenter at the level of the greater wing of the sphenoid bone, which they divided into three thirds (medial, middle, and lateral) [18]. We suggest our own classification system derived from the previous schemes. Our proposed classification system successively takes into account the general morphology of the meningioma, its epicenter in the sphenoid wing, and the tumor invasion of specific anatomical regions and structures (**Figure 4**). These three main parameters are intended to assist in the surgical strategy planning by helping surgical teams determine the anatomical targets, how to reach them, and how to decompress them.

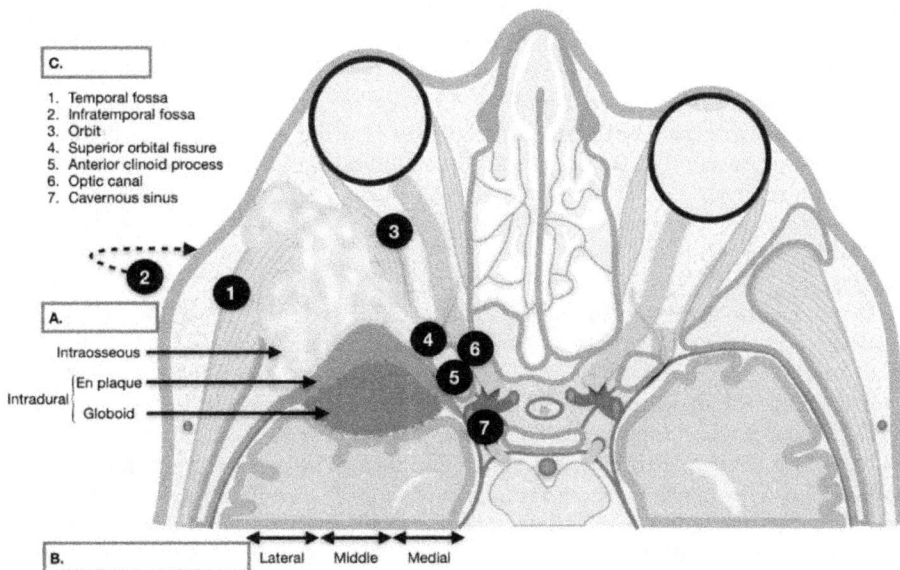

Figure 4.
Classification of spheno-orbital meningiomas according to their morphology (a), sphenoid wing epicenter (b), and specific extensions (c).

7. Surgical technique

7.1 Positioning of the patient and general settings

The patient is placed in a supine position with the head rotated 30° to the contralateral side and fixed in a three-pin Mayfield head-holder. The neck is slightly extended to 15°, as is done for a classical pterional approach. Neuronavigation is used to delineate the craniotomy and skin incision. We recommend using millimeter slices of the bone window of the CT scan for registration, to both highlight bone tumor extension and increase the accuracy of this technique [19, 20]. The CT scan is then merged with the MRI, including the gadolinium-enhanced 3D T1-weighted sequence, for intra- and extracranial tumor extensions (**Figure 4**). A paraumbilical field is prepared and draped to harvest abdominal fat for closure if needed.

7.2 Extracranial steps

The frontotemporal arciform incision starts 1 cm in front of the tragus, with the medial extent adjusted to the size of the surgical target. The scalp is progressively elevated in one layer and reclined forward, preserving the pericranial tissue for dural repair at the time of closure. A standard interfascial dissection is performed over the anterior quarter of the temporal muscle in order to spare the frontotemporal branches of the facial nerve [21, 22]. The orbital rim and zygomatic arch are progressively exposed in a subperiosteal manner. The temporal muscle is incised along the lateral orbital rim, along the superior temporal line, and at its posterior part along the skin incision. Retrograde dissection of the temporal muscle is performed using a cutting spatula from anterior to posterior and from inferior to superior in order to preserve the deep vascularization and innervation of the muscle and thus prevent postoperative atrophy [23]. Tumor-infiltrating of the muscle (1.) temporal fossa extension) must be resected at this stage. If the infratemporal fossa is invaded by the meningioma (2.) infratemporal fossa extension), the zygomatic arch must be cut anteriorly and posteriorly, maintaining its attachment to the masseter muscle, in order to recline the temporal muscle downwards as much as possible. This optional step facilitates resection of the tumor portion located in the infratemporal fossa, with particular attention to the mandibular nerve exiting the foramen ovale. In cases of major invasion of this location, the collaboration of an ear, nose, and throat surgeon is required.

7.3 Cranial steps

Depending on the extension of the intraosseous portion of the SOM, either a classical pterional craniotomy or a more complex orbitozygomatic approach is performed [24]. Guided by neuronavigation, the tumor-infiltrated bone must be resected as completely as possible using a high-speed drill and rongeurs, without overlooking the craniotomy part. The lateral wall and the roof of the orbit are drilled, initially respecting the periorbita (**Figure 5**). The intraorbital tumor extension (3.) mostly remains extraconal and can therefore be easily removed once the orbit is correctly opened. Nevertheless, the periorbit must be longitudinally opened and resected in cases of intraconal invasion [25]. If the tumor adheres too much to the cranial nerves, it is recommended to leave a residue in place to avoid postoperative deficits. The drilling continues medially at the level of the greater and lesser wings of the sphenoid bone, opening the SOF (4.), and inferiorly at the level of the floor of the middle cranial fossa, opening the foramens rotundum and ovale if necessary. With the involvement of the ACP (5.) and the invasion of the optic canal

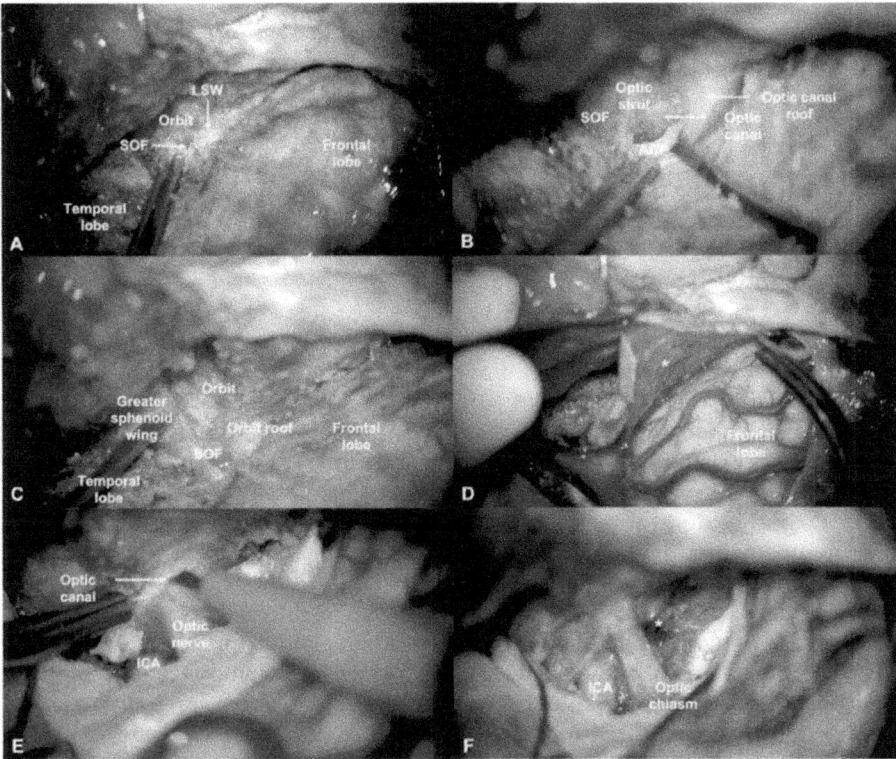

Figure 5.
Intraoperative views of the resection of a left sphenoid-orbital meningioma with invasion of the anterior clinoid process (ACP), optic canal, and orbit. (a) Left pterional approach with drilling of the lesser sphenoid wing (LSW) and lateral wall of the orbit, in order to open the superior orbital fissure (SOF). The orbito-temporal periosteal fold is then identified at the external part of the SOF and divided to optimize the retraction of the frontal and temporal lobes and expose the contours of the ACP. (b) The final step of the extradural resection of the ACP. The LSW, optic strut, and roof of the optic canal were drilled before resecting the bony content inside the ACP. A thin shell of bony contour is preserved in order to remove the clinoid tip en bloc. (c) Once the drilling is completed, the orbit is properly exposed in continuity with the SOF and optic canal which have been opened. (d) The dura mater is opened in an arciform fashion, revealing the intradural portion of the meningioma (asterisk). (e) The dura mater of the optic canal is gently opened with a fine scalpel to remove the tumor fragments compressing the optic nerve at this level. (f) At the end of the procedure, the chiasma and the two optic nerves are correctly exposed. The coagulated portion of the dura mater at the level of the tuberculum sellae can be seen (asterisk; Simpson grade 2 resection).

(6.), an extradural anterior clinoidectomy, which is carried out under magnification and constant irrigation, must be performed to optimize the decompression of the ON and prevent thermic lesions [26]. This step also allows the surgeon to extradurally split the lateral wall of the CS (7.) when there is a tumor at this level, in order to improve the devascularization of the meningioma.

7.4 Intradural steps

The dura mater is opened in a curvilinear fashion and the intradural portion of the tumor is progressively resected using conventional microsurgical methods, alternating debulking and peripheral dissection from the brain parenchyma and vessels. An additional dural incision directed medially toward the optic canal may cautiously be performed to complete the extradural anterior clinoidectomy. Once the optic canal has been widely opened intradurally (**Figure 5**), the tumor fragments at this level can be easily removed using a small blunt hook.

Complete resection is not always possible due to true intracavernous invasion (as opposed to a simple extension to the lateral wall) or excessive tumor adherence in the SOF or optic canal. In such situations, the key is to optimally decompress the ON so that the residual tumor can later be effectively treated with radiation therapy. The radiosensitivity of the ON justifies the creation of a safety zone around it, in order to avoid deleterious iatrogenic irradiation during radiation treatment. It is essential to preserve the function of the cranial nerves as much as possible, as their postoperative recovery is often uncertain.

7.5 Closure and reconstruction

If the ethmoidal or sphenoidal sinuses are open during the extradural steps, either autologous fat or a temporal muscle graft should be harvested to plug the defect, depending on the size of the opening (for example, the muscle should be used for a small aperture of a pneumatized ACP and fat should be used for a large sinus opening secondary to intranasal tumor invasion). A synthetic fibrin sealant may be used in addition to these measures to prevent postoperative cerebrospinal fluid leakage. The dural and periorbital defects are ideally managed using a vascularized and pedicled pericranial graft that is rotated over the orbit. Alternative solutions include using the temporal fascia or synthetic dura patches. Finally, the remaining dead space left by the tumor removal can be filled with a fat graft.

Bone reconstruction for SOM is often more complex than for other meningiomas due to the extensive bony resection, which sometimes involves the superior and lateral orbital rims. Various options are available to perform cranioplasty and obtain a satisfactory cosmetic result. If the orbital margins are intact, the healthy part of the craniotomy can be replaced using grids that are cut to a suitable shape and serve as anchor points for the reinsertion of the temporal muscle. For larger defects, hydroxyapatite cement can be shaped easily. A custom-made polymethylmethacrylate or polyetheretherketone (PEEK) prosthesis can be ordered before the procedure, especially when the orbital rims are planned to be resected. The design of the prosthesis can also compensate for temporal muscle atrophy by incorporating an increased thickening at the level of the temporal fossa. Trimming of the edges of the prosthesis is often required to perfectly match the craniotomy. The zygomatic osteotomy must be reattached with standard plates before reinserting the temporal muscle and suturing the scalp in layers according to the usual technique.

8. Complications and postoperative care

The first postoperative night is ideally spent in an intensive care unit, so that the patient can be closely monitored, and any respiratory, hemodynamic, or neurological failures can be detected at an early stage, particularly in the event of a surgical site hematoma. Most postoperative complications of SOM are related to the cranial nerves affected by the tumor. In their meta-analysis of retrospective series of operated SOM, Fisher *et al.* summarized the incidence of occurrence of these complications [12]. Ophthalmoplegia was frequent (16%) and mainly related to oculomotor nerves damage (oculomotor III 11%; trochlear IV 2%; abducens VI 6%; not specified 13%). In addition, ptosis or diplopia (neuropathic or restrictive) was observed in 17% of cases each. Regarding the optic nerve, visual field loss was described in 4% of cases, while visual acuity was decreased in 9%, and blindness was reported in 3% of cases. Trigeminal hypoesthesia was the most frequent complication (19%); in contrast, facial paralysis was rare (4%). Regarding complications related to the brain, the incidence of epilepsy was estimated to be 8%, while motor and phasic deficits, or diabetes insipidus were uncommon. Enophthalmos and cerebrospinal fluid leaks were encountered in 5% of cases each. Meningitis occurred in 7% and wound infections occurred in 3% of cases, which is consistent with the general rate of infection in cranial surgery, which was reported to be 9% [27]. Finally, pulmonary embolism was diagnosed in 4% of the patients who underwent an operation for SOM.

9. Postoperative course

9.1 Visual function

In most cases, SOM surgery stabilizes or improves visual function. In a large retrospective study of 130 patients, Terrier *et al.* demonstrated improvement in 45% of cases, stabilization in 39%, and worsening in 16% [28]. Fisher *et al.* highlighted in their meta-analysis that visual acuity and visual field were stabilized or improved in 91% and 87% of cases, respectively [12]. However, these encouraging results must be put into perspective, since improvement does not mean a complete restoration of visual function. Anatomically, invasion of the optic canal is associated with severe visual impairment both preoperatively and postoperatively [29], and tumor extension to the periorbit appears to be a negative predictive factor for visual acuity [8]. Therefore, it is essential to propose surgery to patients with SOM as soon as the optic pathways are threatened by the tumor, so that they can be optimally decompressed.

Regarding oculomotion, the reporting of results is generally less detailed, but seems to indicate a long-term improvement of the preoperative symptomatology that could reach 96% (although the degree of this improvement was not specified) [12]. Postoperative oculomotor deficits are frequent, varying from 8 to 68% depending on the series, but they recover in the majority of cases and persist in only 0–17% of cases [6, 11, 30, 31].

9.2 Proptosis

Proptosis, the most common sign encountered in patients with SOM, may be explained by different, yet interrelated, factors. From a mechanical point of view, the bony involvement of the orbital walls and the intraorbital tumor extension exert a direct mass effect on the eyeball. From a vascular point of view, the meningioma invasion of the SOF is responsible for a decrease in venous drainage and subsequently exacerbates the proptosis by increasing the intraorbital venous engorgement [32, 33]. This multifactorial physiopathology may explain the varied results from retrospective clinical series, which report improvements ranging from 50 to 100% [34–39]. Thus, if mechanical compression is relieved by surgical opening of the orbit and resection of the intraorbital portion of the tumor, exophthalmos will certainly improve. Nevertheless, it is rare that the proptosis recovers completely, likely due to persistent disturbances of venous drainage and potential trophic disorders of the oculomotor muscles. Removal of the periorbit appears to have a beneficial effect and seems to be a key factor in reducing proptosis [29].

9.3 Oncological outcome

The quality of surgical resection of meningiomas, assessed by Simpson's grading system, remains an important prognostic factor in the evolution of these tumors, regardless of the histological subtypes considered [40, 41]. Gross total resection, defined as Simpson grade I to III, is achieved in 25–70% of SOM cases depending on the series [34, 42–44]. Given the complex anatomy of the spheno-orbital region, Simpson grade I or II resections are rarely feasible without risking the induction of cranial nerve deficits, especially at the level of the orbital apex, SOF, and CS [43]. In this context, the current trend is strongly in favor of symptom-oriented surgery rather than radical surgery, targeting optic nerve decompression to improve visual function, and intraorbital tumor resection to reduce proptosis [30, 32].

Histologically, SOMs are commonly World Health Organization (WHO) grade I tumors (77–100%, depending on the series), with the meningothelial subtype being the most frequent [11, 13, 28, 43]. Although much less frequent, WHO grade II (atypical) or III (anaplastic) meningiomas may be encountered, together representing 11% of the cases in the retrospective series presented by Belinsky *et al.* Moreover, the authors highlighted the strong correlation between WHO grading, Ki67 proliferation index, and clinical progression [45]. Thus, WHO grade II and III meningiomas, which are associated with an aggressive clinical course and high recurrence rate compared to WHO grade I tumors, have Ki67 proliferation indices that proportionally predict their behavior (14.9 and 58.3, respectively). When considering only WHO grade I SOM, a Ki67 index $\geq$3.3 is associated with a higher risk of recurrence. Comparing these different histological subgroups, Agi *et al.* reported a recurrence rate of 22% in the WHO grade I tumors and 50% in the WHO grade II tumors, with a mean follow-up of 57 months [46].

The highly variable recurrence rate of SOM in the scientific literature, ranging from 10 to 56%, is likely due to differences in the follow-up duration [34, 47–49]. Indeed, the risk of recurrence logically increases with the duration of follow-up (6% at 3 years and 46% at 6 years after the intervention) [28].

The role and timing of radiation therapy remain a matter of debate for meningiomas in general and SOM in particular. However, experts (Response Assessment in Neuro-Oncology Committee) agree on the importance of using adjuvant radiotherapy for WHO grade III meningiomas, regardless of the quality of surgical resection [40]. For WHO grade II meningiomas, the European Association of Neuro-Oncology guidelines recommends observation or fractioned radiotherapy in cases of gross total resection and fractioned radiotherapy in cases of subtotal resection [16]. For WHO grade I meningiomas, simple observation is indicated after gross total resection, and stereotactic radiosurgery or fractioned radiotherapy may be proposed after subtotal resection. We suggest radiological monitoring of the tumor residue for subtotal resections of WHO grade I meningiomas initially. Stereotactic radiosurgery is then justified in cases of objective progression. Cases of meningiomas of WHO grade II or III must be discussed in a collegial manner in a multidisciplinary consultation meeting.

10. Conclusion

Spheno-orbital meningiomas are usually slow-growing skull base tumors revealed by proptosis or visual impairment. They typically present with significant tumoral spheno-orbital hyperostosis and a globoid or *en plaque* intradural portion. As their epicenter is located at the level of the lesser and greater sphenoid wings, they progressively extend to the temporal and infratemporal fossae, orbit, anterior clinoid process, and cavernous sinus, compromising the integrity of the optic canal, the superior orbital fissure, and the cranial nerves passing through. The reference treatment is currently optimal surgical resection after complete ophthalmological examination and radiological evaluation by MRI and CT scan. Although the risk of recurrence appears to be clearly correlated with the quality of the surgical resection, in cases with excessive meningioma adherence to critical anatomical structures, the removal of the tumor must be restricted in order to limit the comorbidities related to induced cranial nerves deficits. Radiation therapy is a safe option after surgery for recurrent or aggressive meningiomas.

Abbreviations

ACP	Anterior clinoid process
CS	Cavernous sinus
CT	Computed tomography
MRI	Magnetic resonance imaging
OCT	Optical coherence tomography
ON	Optic nerve
SOF	Superior orbital fissure
SOM	Spheno-orbital meningioma
WHO	World Health Organization

Author details

Guillaume Baucher[1,2*], Lucas Troude[1,2] and Pierre-Hugues Roche[1,2]

1 Assistance Publique-Hôpitaux de Marseille, Hôpital Universitaire Nord, Neurochirurgie adulte, Marseille, France

2 Aix-Marseille Université, Marseille, France

*Address all correspondence to: guillaume.baucher@ap-hm.fr

IntechOpen

References

[1] Cushing H. The menigiomas (dural endotheliomas): Their source, and favoured seats of origin. Brain. 1922;**45**:282-316. DOI: 10.1093/brain/45.2.282

[2] Cushing H, Eisenhardt L. Meningiomas. Their classification, regional behaviour. Life history, and surgical end results. Bulletin of the Medical Library Association. 1938;**27**:185-185

[3] Di Cristofori A, Del Bene M, Locatelli M, Boggio F, Ercoli G, Ferrero S, et al. Meningioma and bone hyperostosis: Expression of bone stimulating factors and review of the literature. World Neurosurgery. 2018;**115**:e774-e781. DOI: 10.1016/j.wneu.2018.04.176

[4] Pieper DR, Al-Mefty O, Hanada Y, Buechner D. Hyperostosis associated with meningioma of the Cranial Base: Secondary changes or tumor invasion. Neurosurgery. 1999;**44**:742-746. DOI: 10.1097/00006123-199904000-00028

[5] De Jesús O, Toledo MM. Surgical management of meningioma en plaque of the sphenoid ridge. Surgical Neurology. 2001;**55**:265-269. DOI: 10.1016/S0090-3019(01)00440-2

[6] Ringel F, Cedzich C, Schramm J. Microsurgical technique and results of a series of 63 spheno-orbital meningiomas. Operative Neurosurgery. 2007;**60**:214-222. DOI: 10.1227/01.NEU.0000255415.47937.1A

[7] Kiyofuji S, Casabella AM, Graffeo CS, Perry A, Garrity JA, Link MJ. Sphenoorbital meningioma: A unique skull base tumor. Surgical technique and results. Journal of Neurosurgery. 2020;**133**:1044-1051. DOI: 10.3171/2019.6.JNS191158

[8] Forster M-T, Daneshvar K, Senft C, Seifert V, Marquardt G. Sphenoorbital meningiomas: Surgical management and outcome. Neurological Research. 2014;**36**:695-700. DOI: 10.1179/1743132814Y.0000000329

[9] Bondy M, Lee LB. Epidemiology and etiology of intracranial meningiomas: A review. Journal of Neuro-Oncology. 1996;**29**:197-205. DOI: 10.1007/BF00165649

[10] Claus EB, Bondy ML, Schildkraut JM, Wiemels JL, Wrensch M, Black PM. Epidemiology of intracranial meningioma. Neurosurgery. 2005;**57**:1088-1095. DOI: 10.1227/01.NEU.0000188281.91351.B9

[11] Menon SOS, Anand D, Menon G. Spheno-orbital meningiomas: Optimizing visual outcome. Journal of Neurosciences in Rural Practice. 2020;**11**:385-394. DOI: 10.1055/s-0040-1709270

[12] Fisher FL, Zamanipoor Najafabadi AH, Schoones JW, Genders SW, Furth WR. Surgery as a safe and effective treatment option for spheno-orbital meningioma: A systematic review and meta-analysis of surgical techniques and outcomes. Acta Ophthalmologica. 2021;**99**:26-36. DOI: 10.1111/aos.14517

[13] Apra C, Roblot P, Alkhayri A, Le Guérinel C, Polivka M, Chauvet D. Female gender and exogenous progesterone exposition as risk factors for spheno-orbital meningiomas. Journal of Neuro-Oncology. 2020;**149**:95-101. DOI: 10.1007/s11060-020-03576-8

[14] Dolecek TA, Propp JM, Stroup NE, Kruchko C. CBTRUS statistical report: Primary brain and central nervous system tumors diagnosed in the United

States in 2005-2009. Neuro-Oncology. 2012;**14**:v1-v49. DOI: 10.1093/neuonc/nos218

[15] DeMonte F, McDermott MW, Al-Mefty O. Al-Mefty's Meningiomas. Stuttgart: Georg Thieme Verlag; 2011

[16] Goldbrunner R, Minniti G, Preusser M, Jenkinson MD, Sallabanda K, Houdart E, et al. EANO guidelines for the diagnosis and treatment of meningiomas. The Lancet Oncology. 2016;**17**:e383-e391. DOI: 10.1016/S1470-2045(16)30321-7

[17] Roser F, Nakamura M, Jacobs C, Vorkapic P, Samii M. Sphenoid wing meningiomas with osseous involvement. Surgical Neurology. 2005;**64**:37-43. DOI: 10.1016/j.surneu.2004.08.092

[18] Kong D-S, Kim YH, Hong C-K. Optimal indications and limitations of endoscopic transorbital superior eyelid surgery for spheno-orbital meningiomas. Journal of Neurosurgery. 2021;**134**:1472-1479. DOI: 10.3171/2020.3.JNS20297

[19] Marcus H, Schwindack C, Santarius T, Mannion R, Kirollos R. Image-guided resection of spheno-orbital skull-base meningiomas with predominant intraosseous component. Acta Neurochirurgica. 2013;**155**:981-988. DOI: 10.1007/s00701-013-1662-8

[20] Poggi S, Pallotta S, Russo S, Gallina P, Torresin A, Bucciolini M. Neuronavigation accuracy dependence on CT and MR imaging parameters: A phantom-based study. Physics in Medicine & Biology. 2003;**48**:2199-2216. DOI: 10.1088/0031-9155/48/14/311

[21] Baucher G, Bernard F, Graillon T, Dufour H. Interfascial approach for pterional craniotomy: technique and adjustments to prevent cosmetic complications. Acta Neurochirurgica. 2019;**161**(11):2353-2357. DOI: 10.1007/s00701-019-04058-1

[22] Yasargil MG. Microneurosurgery: Microsurgical Anatomy of the Basal Cisterns and Vessels of the Brain, Diagnostic Studies, General Operative Techniques and Pathological Considerations of the Intracranial Aneurysms. 1st ed., 21621st ed. New York, New York, United States: Thieme Medical Publishers; 1985

[23] Oikawa S, Mizuno M, Muraoka S, Kobayashi S. Retrograde dissection of the temporalis muscle preventing muscle atrophy for pterional craniotomy. Journal of Neurosurgery. 1996;**84**:297-299

[24] Zabramski JM, Kiriş T, Sankhla SK, Cabiol J, Spetzler RF. Orbitozygomatic craniotomy: Technical note. Journal of Neurosurgery. 1998;**89**:336-341. DOI: 10.3171/jns.1998.89.2.0336

[25] Troude L, Bernard F, Roche P-H. The medial orbito-frontal approach for orbital tumors: A how I do it. Acta Neurochirurgica. 2017;**159**:2223-2227. DOI: 10.1007/s00701-017-3319-5

[26] Troude L, Bernard F, Baucher G, De La Rosa Morilla S, Roche P-H. Extradural resection of the anterior clinoid process: How I do it. Neuro-Chirurgie. 2017;**63**:336-340. DOI: 10.1016/j.neuchi.2017.03.001

[27] Boissonneau S, Tsiaremby M, Peyriere H, Graillon T, Farah K, Fuentes S, et al. Post-operative complications in cranial and spine neurosurgery: a prospective observational study. Journal of Neurosurgical Sciences. March 2021. Available from: https://www.minervamedica.it/en/journals/neurosurgical-sciences/article.php?cod=R38Y9999N00A21031101. DOI: 10.23736/S0390-5616.21.05083-9

[28] Terrier L-M, Bernard F, Fournier H-D, Morandi X, Velut S, Hénaux P-L, et al. Spheno-orbital meningiomas

surgery: Multicenter management study for complex extensive tumors. World Neurosurgery. 2018;**112**:e145-e156. DOI: 10.1016/j.wneu.2017.12.182

[29] Yannick N, Patrick F, Samuel M, Erwan F, Pierre-Jean P, Michel J, et al. Predictive factors for visual outcome after resection of spheno-orbital meningiomas: A long-term review. Acta Ophthalmologica. 2012;**90**:e663-e665. DOI: 10.1111/j.1755-3768.2012.02419.x

[30] Freeman JL, Davern MS, Oushy S, Sillau S, Ormond DR, Youssef AS, et al. Spheno-orbital meningiomas: A 16-year surgical experience. World Neurosurgery. 2017;**99**:369-380. DOI: 10.1016/j.wneu.2016.12.063

[31] Shrivastava RK, Sen C, Costantino PD, Della Rocca R. Sphenoorbital meningiomas: Surgical limitations and lessons learned in their long-term management. Journal of Neurosurgery. 2005;**103**:491-497. DOI: 10.3171/jns.2005.103.3.0491

[32] Saeed P, van Furth WR, Tanck M, Kooremans F, Freling N, Streekstra GI, et al. Natural history of spheno-orbital meningiomas. Acta Neurochirurgica. 2011;**153**:395-402. DOI: 10.1007/s00701-010-0878-0

[33] Scarone P, Leclerq D, Héran F, Robert G. Long-term results with exophthalmos in a surgical series of 30 sphenoorbital meningiomas: Clinical article. Journal of Neurosurgery. 2009;**111**:1069-1077. DOI: 10.3171/2009.1.JNS081263

[34] Boari N, Gagliardi F, Spina A, Bailo M, Franzin A, Mortini P. Management of spheno-orbital en plaque meningiomas: Clinical outcome in a consecutive series of 40 patients. British Journal of Neurosurgery. 2013;**27**:84-90. DOI: 10.3109/02688697.2012.709557

[35] Cannon PS, Rutherford SA, Richardson PL, King A,

Leatherbarrow B. The surgical management and outcomes for Spheno-orbital meningiomas: A 7-year review of multi-disciplinary practice. Orbit. 2009;**28**:371-376. DOI: 10.3109/01676830903104645

[36] Civit T, Freppel S. Méningiomes sphéno-orbitaires. Neuro-Chirurgie. 2010;**56**:124-131. DOI: 10.1016/j.neuchi.2010.02.022

[37] Franquet N, Pellerin P, Dhellemmes P, Defoort-Dhellemmes S. Manifestations ophtalmologiques des méningiomes sphéno-orbitaires. Journal Français d'Ophtalmologie. 2009;**32**:16-19. DOI: 10.1016/j.jfo.2008.11.005

[38] Mirone G, Chibbaro S, Schiabello L, Tola S, George B. En plaque sphenoid wing meningiomas: Recurrence factors and surgical strategy in a series of 71 patients. Operative Neurosurgery. 2009;**65**:100-109. DOI: 10.1227/01.NEU.0000345652.19200.D5

[39] Talacchi A, De Carlo A, D'Agostino A, Nocini P. Surgical management of ocular symptoms in spheno-orbital meningiomas. Is orbital reconstruction really necessary? Neurosurgical Review. 2014;**37**:301-310. DOI: 10.1007/s10143-014-0517-y

[40] Rogers L, Barani I, Chamberlain M, Kaley TJ, McDermott M, Raizer J, et al. Meningiomas: Knowledge base, treatment outcomes, and uncertainties. A RANO review. Journal of Neurosurgery. 2015;**122**:4-23. DOI: 10.3171/2014.7.JNS131644

[41] Simpson D. The recurrence of intracranial meningiomas after surgical treatment. Journal of Neurology, Neurosurgery & Psychiatry. 1957;**20**:22-39. DOI: 10.1136/jnnp.20.1.22

[42] Honig S, Trantakis C, Frerich B, Sterker I, Schober R, Meixensberger J. Spheno-orbital meningiomas: Outcome after microsurgical treatment: A

clinical review of 30 cases. Neurological Research. 2010;**32**: 314-325. DOI: 10.1179/016164109X1246 4612122614

[43] Masalha W, Heiland DH, Steiert C, Krüger MT, Schnell D, Scheiwe C, et al. Progression-free survival, prognostic factors, and surgical outcome of Spheno-orbital meningiomas. Frontiers in Oncology. 2021;**11**:672228. DOI: 10.3389/fonc.2021.672228

[44] Oya S, Sade B, Lee JH. Sphenoorbital meningioma: Surgical technique and outcome: Clinical article. Journal of Neurosurgery. 2011;**114**:1241-1249. DOI: 10.3171/2010.10.JNS101128

[45] Belinsky I, Murchison AP, Evans JJ, Andrews DW, Farrell CJ, Casey JP, et al. Spheno-orbital meningiomas: An analysis based on World Health Organization classification and Ki-67 proliferative index. Ophthalmic Plastic & Reconstructive Surgery. 2018;**34**:143-150. DOI: 10.1097/ IOP.0000000000000904

[46] Agi J, Badilla J, Steinke D, Mitha AP, Weis E. The Alberta standardized orbital technique in the management of spheno-orbital meningiomas. European Journal of Ophthalmology. 2020;**31**(5): 112067212096033. DOI: 10.1177/ 1120672120960332

[47] Heufelder MJ, Sterker I, Trantakis C, Schneider J-P, Meixensberger J, Hemprich A, et al. Reconstructive and ophthalmologic outcomes following resection of Spheno-orbital meningiomas. Ophthalmic Plastic & Reconstructive Surgery. 2009;**25**:223-226. DOI: 10.1097/IOP.0b013e3181a1f345

[48] Mariniello G, Maiuri F, Strianese D, Donzelli R, Iuliano A, Tranfa F, et al. Spheno-orbital meningiomas: Surgical approaches and outcome according to the Intraorbital tumor extent. Central European Neurosurgery-Zentralblatt für Neurochirurgie. 2008;**69**:175-181. DOI: 10.1055/s-2008-1077077

[49] Sandalcioglu IE, Gasser T, Mohr C, Stolke D, Wiedemayer H. Sphenoorbital meningiomas: Interdisciplinary surgical approach, resectability and long-term results. Journal of Cranio-Maxillofacial Surgery. 2005;**33**:260-266. DOI: 10.1016/j.jcms.2005.01.013

Chapter 4

Surgery of Meningiomas of the Anterior Clinoid Process

Oleksandr Voznyak and Nazarii Hryniv

Abstract

Sphenoid wing meningiomas account for 11%-20% of all intracranial meningiomas, whereas meningiomas of the anterior clinoid process comprise about 34.0–43.9%. Assignment of these cranio-basal tumors to a separate group is due to the parasellar location and challenges in their surgical removal, mainly because of its anatomical syntopy: compression of the optic nerve, carotid artery inclusion, and invasion to the cavernous sinus. This chapter consists of the combination of current knowledge and our experience in understanding, diagnosis, surgical strategy, and complication avoidance with these tumors.

Keywords: sphenoid wing meningioma, classification, anterior clinoid process, clinoidectomy, parasellar syntopy, pterional approach, fronto-lateral approach, skull base

1. Introduction

Meningiomas are the most common primary intracranial tumors accounting for 20% of all intracranial neoplasms. Sphenoid wing meningiomas (SWM) account for 11%-20% of all intracranial meningiomas. Meningiomas of the anterior clinoid process (MAC) comprise about 34.0–43.9% of all sphenoid wing meningiomas. There is female prevalence among patients [1–3].

The challenges start with the definition of MAC. From the early beginning, H. Cushing and Eisenhardt in 1938 were the first to divide SWM into globoid tumors with a nodular shape and en plaque tumors, which are flat and spread along the sphenoid wing [2]. The globoid tumors were then categorized into lateral, middle, and medial. The last group could be classified as MAC. In accordance with Al-Mefti, MAC was classified into 3 groups according to the side of their origin on the surface of the clinoid process. First group meningiomas arise from the subclinoidal dura at the most proximal point of intradural entry of the internal carotid artery, before the carotid enters into the arachnoidal cisternal space. The second group clinoidal meningiomas originates from the superolateral aspect of the anterior clinoid process. The third group originates from the region of the optic foramen and extends into the optic canal [1, 4]. Many authors consider this classification hard to apply in daily practice. Russell & Benjamin took into account the invasion of the tumor into the lesser sphenoid wing and spread into the cavernous sinus [3]. Both parameters have great practical significance in surgical approach planning [5].

The exclusion method is also useful to identify the MAC. All paraoptic meningiomas such as tuberculum sella, diaphragm, cavernous sinus, planum sphenoidale, as well as spheno-orbital are recognizable with their specific findings [6, 7, 9]. We

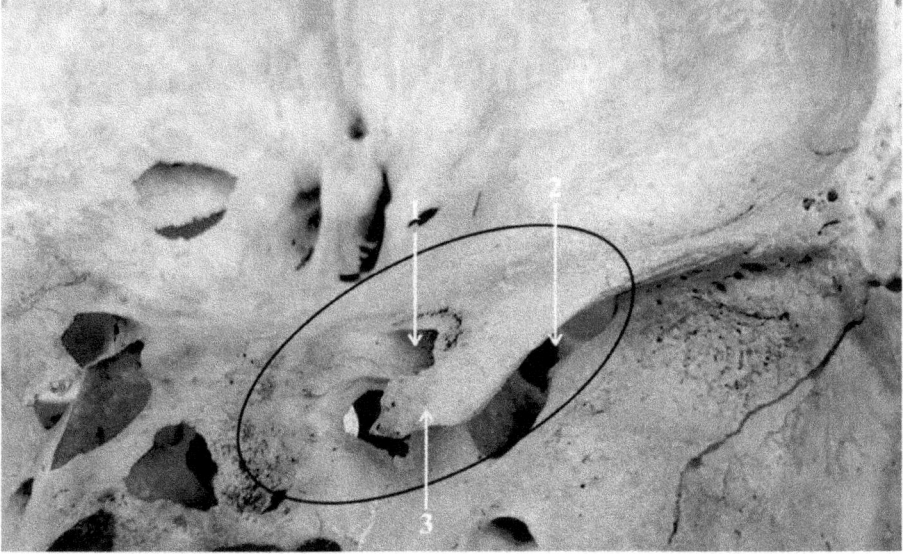

Figure 1.
Anterior clinoid bone anatomy, right side. 1 – Optic canal; 2 – Superior orbital fissure; 3 – Anterior clinoid process.

consider the presence of the anterior clinoid process in the center of the tumor bone attachment to be the main feature of clinoidal meningiomas (**Figure 1**). The second apparent peculiarity is the paramedian location of the tumor and consequently the displaced ipsilateral optic nerve, III nerve, and the ICA toward the midline [8–10].

2. Anatomical aspects

Anterior clinoid process (ACP) is tetrahedron in shape with the apex projected medio-posteriorly. Medially, it forms a superolateral wall of the optic canal. The optic strut is the posterior root of the ACP. Anteriorly it continues with the medial aspect of the sphenoid ridge.

As a rule, the process comprises the bony cortex. However, its pneumatization and bony connections could be variable and attention should be paid before the planned removal.

The removal of the process reveals the 2-6 cm long clinoid space [10]. The dural layer between this space and ACP is the deep extension from the roof of the cavernous sinus and covers the inferior surface of the clinoid process. Medially, this layer extends to surround the ICA as the proximal dural ring and turns upward along the clinoid segment of the ICA to fuse with the distal dural ring. The dural connection between the 3rd nerve and the lateral aspect of the distal dural ring is called the carotico-oculomotor membrane. From the inferolateral aspect of the ACP, the neural bundle consisting of 3rd, 4th, 6th and three branches of the ophthalmic nerve are running. Thus, manipulation in the inferior direction exposes these structures to danger and should be avoided [11, 12]. Meningiomas usually invade the outer (temporal) dural leaf and rarely spread to dura propria (DP), so the separation of dural leaves during surgery provides an increased removal rate as well as better visualization of anatomical structures [13, 14].

C2 and C3 segments of ICA (Bouthillier nomenclature) are traversing the horizontal and vertical portion of the carotid canal in the petrous bone. The cavernous

C4 segment is forming a carotid siphon, surrounded by venous plexus. This portion ends with the dural entrance through the proximal dural ring. The number of veins surrounding the clinoid meningioma is not constant. The superficial middle cerebral vein (SMCV) drains the lateral part of the cerebral hemisphere into the cavernous sinus (CS) directly by penetrating its lateral wall and indirectly through the sphenoparietal sinus or through the latero-cavernous sinus. Sphenoparietal sinus runs medially just below the lesser sphenoid wing to empty into the anterior part of the CS [15, 16].

3. Syntopy

Understanding of ACP syntopy with surrounding anatomical structures is extremely important for surgical dissection and anterior clinoidectomy during surgery. The base of the process forms the lateral and lower walls of the optic canal, the medial surface forms the ICA canal, and the lateral surface and optic strut are the parts of the upper medial wall of the upper orbit (**Figure 1**). Thus, ACP is located between the canal of the optic nerve, upper orbital fissure, and ICA canal. Extradural resection of the process provides the access to these bony channels and their content. The clinoidal process also separates two leaves of the dura: dura temporalis (DT) and DP. DP represents the lateral wall of the cavernous sinus and extends from the outer to the inner dural rings, where the ICA penetrates the cavernous sinus. Also, it touches the free edge of the tentorium in posterior divisions, which is fixed to the apex of the ACP [17]. Anteriorly it continues to the layers of the upper orbit. It should be remembered that ACP meningiomas usually invade the outer leaf of the dura and very rarely are spread to the DP. Thus, the separation of the dural leaves during surgery allows exposure of the lateral surface of the ACP and provides consequent visualization of the important anatomical structures of the skull base [17, 18].

After performing extradural clinoidectomy, the optic nerve in the dural sheath could be visualized [19, 20]. The lateral wall of the cavernous sinus and the intracavernous part of the ICA that is passing behind are seen as well. The 3rd nerve is located immediately below the projection of the lower clinoidal edge. The 1st branch of the V nerve passes lower.

Variable pathological anatomy of this area due to tumor growth has to be taken into account. Most clinoid meningiomas invade ACP causing its hyperostotic enlargement [21, 22]. Thus, anterior clinoidectomy is considered the key to the radicality of surgery.

However, there is a group of meningiomas that grows from the superior or superolateral surface of the clinoid without invasion into the ACP and hyperostosis does not exist [23–25]. Complete clinoidectomy is not necessary for this type of MAC.

Intradural syntopy in presence of MAC is much more complex and variable in comparison with extradural peculiarities. Primarily, it is due to the nature of meningioma spread, that has two patterns: expansive and invasive. The first type has a small fixation area and the tumor "wraps" around vessels and nerves. Invasive type spreads along the dura and longitudinally ingrowth into the anatomical structures [26]. In practice, a combination of both types with some predominance is usually seen.

The important tip is to follow the olfactory nerve that always leads to the optic nerve if the last is markedly displaced by the tumor.

A1 segment of ACA and all anterior semicircle of Willis are shifted medially and located on the dorsomedial surface of meningioma. M1 segment of MCA "rolls over" through the dome of the tumor on its upper lateral surface. Special attention to perforating and small branches of the anterior circle of Willis should be paid because of their tight inclusion in the tumor [27]. Sharp dissection is the only possible method to separate them from the tumor.

The oculomotor nerve is displaced dorso-medially and could be encased by neoplasm.

The pituitary stalk itself is not commonly involved in MAC, located on the postero-medial portion of meningioma, and could be separated without difficulties. Although, the superior hypophyseal artery has a variable way and has to be saved to prevent postoperative diabetes insipidus.

4. Diagnosis

Despite the fact that advanced imaging techniques are more accessible and have advantages in certain scenarios, the computed tomography and MRI routine scans remain the standard investigations for patients with MAC [28]. Hyperostosis, bone structures, and anatomical syntopy could be assessed with standard protocols. CT is informative in assessing the bony structures of the skull base, especially anterior clinoid hyperostosis, as well as to determine the presence of petrifications in the tumor. This examination is routinely performed the next day after surgery to control the extent of the tumor removal and exclude the hematoma.

Some features are associated with more aggressive meningiomas and include increased signals on both T1- and T2-weighted MRI, irregular contour, extensive edema, lack of calcifications, central necrosis, and low apparent diffusion coefficient [29]. However, if normal anatomy is variable, the more challenging pathological anatomy influenced by the tumor makes the strategy individual.

Attention should be paid to the tumoral entrapment of the supraclinoid part of the ICA. The ICA is "enveloped" and can *potentially* be dissected from the tumor if the tumor does not invade the bone, CS, and grows expansively in the intracranial direction. Circular encasement of the ICA by the tumor that spreads from the CS along the artery makes its surgical separation almost impossible [30].

Thus, we tend to divide MAC into two main types. The first includes tumors that do not invade the anterior clinoid process and grow expansively into the cranial cavity. Type II meningiomas involve the ACP, spread into the CS, and concentrically entrap the supraclinoid segment of the ICA. There is a sense to separate the second subgroup of tumors: with the penetration to the CS and without it. Anatomical criteria for distribution are demonstrated in **Table 1** and **Figures 2–4**.

	Type I	**Type IIA**	**Type IIB**
Anterior clinoid process hyperostosis	—	+	+
Cavernous sinus invasion	—	—	+
Internal carotid artery entrapment	Shifting / Wrapping	Wrapping / Adhesion	Concentric encasement
Needed clinoidectomy	Partial	Total	Total
Surgical approach	Fronto-lateral* intradural	Pterional extradural	Pterional extradural

*In absence of peritumoral edema.

Table 1.
Criteria for distribution of sphenoid meningiomas.

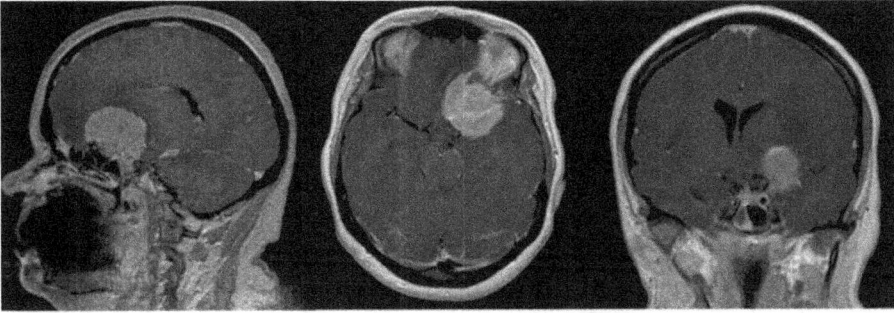

Figure 2.
Type I sphenoid meningioma.

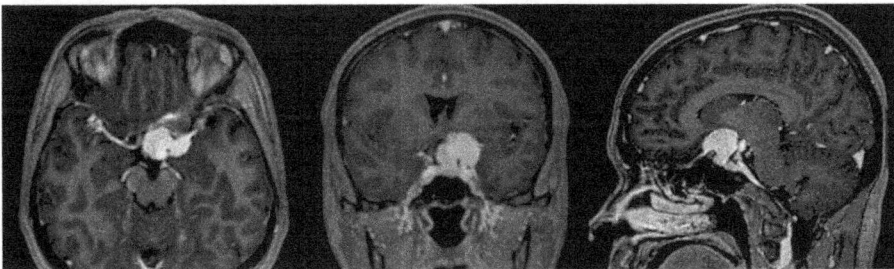

Figure 3.
Type IIA sphenoid meningioma.

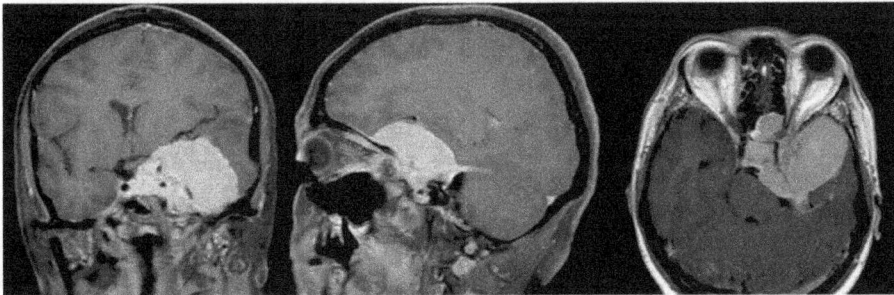

Figure 4.
Type IIB sphenoid meningioma.

Many surgeons recommend performing angiography before surgery to determine the tumor's blood supply and venous features. We totally agree with the expediency of this study, however, we would not insist on the absolute need to conduct it to all patients with this pathology.

5. Surgical approaches

According to the literature, several surgical approaches are used to remove sphenoid meningiomas: subfrontal, fronto-lateral, fronto-temporal intradural, pterional, fronto-temporo-orbito-zygomatic [14, 31, 32]. Eyebrow incision supraorbital keyhole approach (essential modification of the standard frontal-lateral/supraorbital) could be used as well [33]. Recently, several authors have reported their experience using this approach in the management of tumorous lesions around the sellar region [34, 35].

We are using two surgical approaches in our practice: fronto-lateral supraorbital and pterional. The advantages and disadvantages of both approaches are presented in **Table 2.**

In general, the patient's body should be strictly fixated despite the chosen approach to allow the operative field position and angles change. A rigid fixation of the head in the Mayfield or Sugita skull clamp should be used. We have abandoned the use of lumbar drainage to relax the brain during surgery. All surgeries are performed under general anesthesia with artificial lung ventilation.

5.1 Pterional approach

The head is turned away from the side of the craniotomy and the neck should be extended so that malar eminence is at the highest point of the operative field to allow gravity to facilitate brain retraction. The neck should be positioned to avoid excessive compression of jugular veins and the endotracheal tube. Elevation of the head of the bed and ipsilateral shoulder elevation with a pad is used to ensure adequate jugular venous return. The hair is shaved, extending for 3 cm behind the hairline. Skin is incised in a curvilinear fashion from 1 cm anterior to the tragus to the midline. Temporalis muscle is divided by electrocautery and the myocutaneous flap is reflected anteriorly and inferiorly by the subperiosteal dissection with the periosteal elevator and minimal electrocautery, until the root of the zygoma, keyhole, and supraorbital ridge are identified. Posteriorly, the temporalis muscle is retracted for additional temporal exposure.

Adjacent to the Sylvian fissure parts of the frontal and temporal lobes should be widely exposed during the trepanation window formation. The extradural stage includes pterion and lateral orbit drilling. The meningo-orbital band is cut. Dura propria and temporalis are separated from each other. The removal of hyperostotic ACP is impossible without this maneuver. MAC usually involves only temporal dura, thus DP serves as a great orientation layer covering cavernous sinus and protecting its structures during dissection. Intraoperative ultrasound investigation and neuromonitoring should be used during this stage to ensure the ICA and adjacent III and V1 nerves location. Before the intradural stage, it is necessary to visualize the optic nerve in the dural sheath, ICA, and the lateral wall of the cavernous sinus. Arcuate dural incision along the tumoral border allows to use the proximal undamaged dura as brain protection. Incision prolongs to the dura that rostrally covers the optic nerve and then along the upper edge of the cavernous sinus caudally. The edges are connected along the upper part of the cavernous sinus. Mobilized shred is removed together with the adjacent tumor (**Figure 5**).

	Fronto-lateral	**Pterional**
Surgical corridor	Intradural	Extradural
Clinoidectomy	Intradural partial	Extradural
Exposure of optic nerve and internal carotid artery	Intradural after dissection and debulking of tumor	Extradural before the tumor dissection
Meningioma devascularization	During the removal	Mainly before the removal
Need for Sylvian fissure dissection	+	—
Need for cerebral traction	Frontal lobe	Minimal due to protective dura

Table 2.
Advantages and disadvantages of pterional and fronto-lateral approaches.

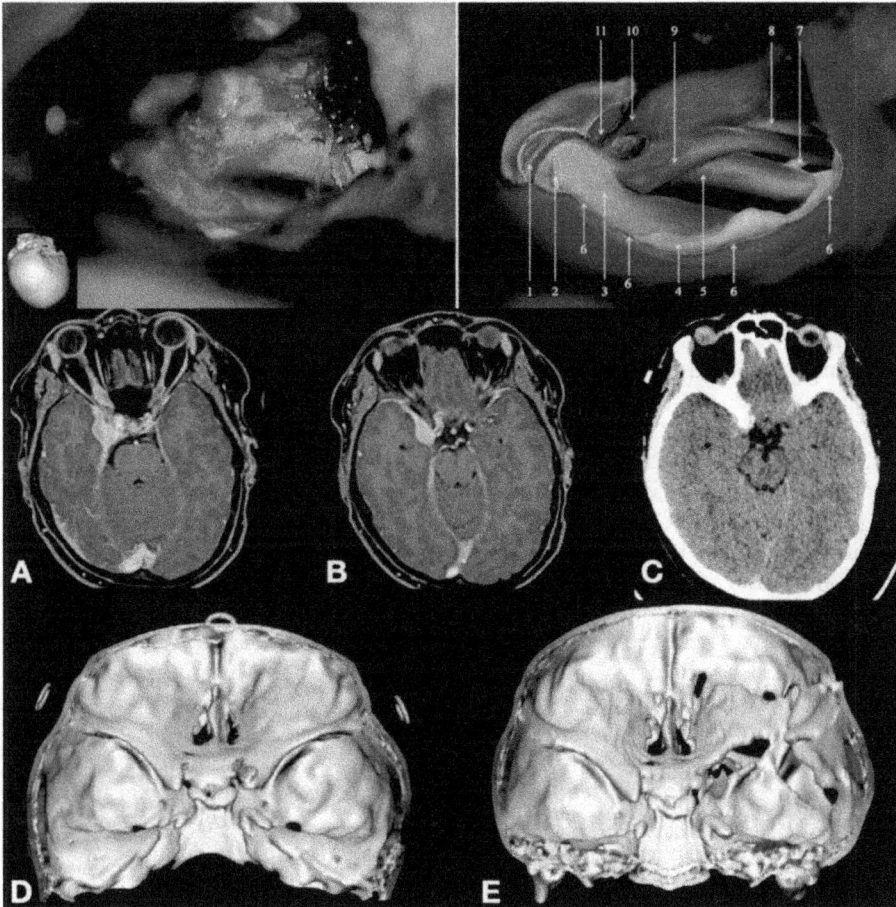

Figure 5.
Final view after tumor removal, right side. 1 – Drilled optic canal 2 – Incised dura around the optic nerve 3 – Optic nerve 4 – Brain tissue 5 – Internal carotid artery 6 – Dural edge 7 – Posterior communicant artery 8 – Oculomotor nerve 9 – Distal dural ring 10 – Superior orbital fissure (connected with optic canal) 11 – Drilled clinoid base; A and B – Preoperative MRI; C – Preoperative CT; D – Preoperative 3D CT bone reconstruction; E – Postoperative 3D CT bone reconstruction.

At this stage, the ON and supraclinoid segment of the ICA could be visualized. Markedly deprived from the blood supply, the tumor is debulked. Incrementally, the tumor is dissected from ON, chiasm, pituitary stalk, 3rd nerve, bran surface, ICA, PCA, ACA, MCA, and their branches in a sharp manner. Wound hermitization could be conducted with fat or vascularized galeo-aponeurotic flap.

5.2 Fronto-lateral supraorbital approach

The position of the patient is on his back. The head is raised and turned by 30° from the approach side. The skin incision is performed along the edge of hair growth. The musculocutaneous flap is directed toward the superciliary arch. Supraorbitally, a bone flap of approximately 5x3 cm is formed. Avoidance of frontal sinus opening is important and the mucous membrane should be dissected from the bone and sutured by atraumatic sutures if opened. Following the arcuate dural incision, CSF aspiration during Sylvian fissure dissection provides the brain's relaxation and wide working space. There is a tendency to avoid using a retractor for the frontal lobe. Even if needed, the use should be as the "brain holder" but not for the forced retraction. Tumor dissection is started from the attachment point and after the ICA, 2nd and 3rd nerves visualization the separation from the basal attachment could be safely ended. Following the main arterial supply deprivation, the tumor usually becomes softer and the volume reduction is effectively conducted. This step allows crucial structures to release. The superior and lateral surface of the anterior clinoid bone as well as the optic nerve roof should be skeletonized by excision of the involved dura. The optic canal is opened necessarily and the anterior clinoid process is drilled within its tumor germination. The procedure is ended with the hermetic dural suturing, fixation of the bone flap, and suturing of the skin.

6. Complication avoidance

Skull base surgery is technically complex and requires special training of the entire neurosurgical team. The procedure should be performed step by step, as each subsequent stage is possible only after the perfect execution of the previous ones. This form of organization as well as applying general principles of craniobasal surgery prevents the majority of surgical complications [36, 37]. Today, mortality after sphenoid wing meningioma surgery does not exceed 1.2% (0.6-1.8%).

In addition to technical aspects, the correct position of the body and head, the presence of neuronavigation and the intraoperative neuromonitoring system accompanied with a well-prepared neurophysiologist are no less important [38, 39]. The confidence with a set of special micro instruments and its appropriate application is crucial. Co-working with anesthesiologists is of great importance in managing the brain edema and consequences of nerves, meninges, and other immediately reactive structures irritation.

The most common complications after the removal of the sphenoid wing meningioma are deterioration of vision, 3rd nerve damage, vascular accidents due to vessels injury, and CSF leakage [36].

6.1 Optic nerve

Visual impairment is usually the first and main symptom and the primary goal of surgery is to preserve and improve the visual function of these patients.

Thus, early extradural visualization following the anterior clinoidectomy and intensive irrigation while drilling to prevent thermal damage is extremely important.

Dissection of the optic nerve sheath, as well as the falciform ligament, allow to explore the nerve in the optic canal, remove the intracanal portion of the tumor, and to ensure the complete ON decompression in the bone canal. Subsequent intracranial dissection from the tumor should be gentle to cause minimal injury of the ON and chiasm.

Early visualization of the ON is challenging in the case of the intradural frontolateral approach as it is covered with a tumor. The fixation point of MAP often extends to the roof of the optic canal. The risk of thermal damage of the optic nerve is high during the attachment site coagulation. We coagulate and separate the meningioma not directly along the basal dura, but retreating a few millimeters into the tumor mass. This maneuver lowers the risk of ON sacrifice. Ophthalmic nerves could serve as a landmark to find the 2nd nerve as I and II nerves as they are always overcrossing.

6.2 Oculomotor nerve

The oculomotor nerve has a low tolerance to any traumatic impact, so the violation of its function is possible even in the absence of direct manipulation with it during surgery. Nevertheless, if the 3rd nerve has not suffered serious traumatic impact intraoperatively, its function will be restored within 1-3 months postoperatively.

In contrast to pterional, the risk of damage to the 3rd nerve is minimal via the fronto-lateral approach. The oculomotor nerve passes directly below the lower edge of the wing, so clinoidectomy and separation of the two dural leaves could be harmful. Attentive dissection of DP and DT along with the plan, adequate irrigation, and coagulation avoidance in this area provide a better chance to pass by troubles.

The intracranial area of the 3rd nerve can be visualized after removal of the germinated basal dura. Sometimes it is appropriate to cut the 3rd nerve meningeal canal, to reach the tumor in the CS.

6.3 Arteries

Detection of the ICA is challenging because it is covered with a tumor. The point is to estimate the character of MAP adhesion to the arterial wall as early as possible. Intimate fusion makes surgical separation impossible because of the risk of arterial wall damage. The so-called "proximal control" proposed by Al-Mefty is not frequently used nowadays. Comparing two approaches in the context of ICA damage risk, the intradural approach is more dangerous because of the need to go through the mass of the tumor to reach the artery wall without having a plan for dissection. In contrast, the extradural approach provides the opportunity to assess the degree of adhesion by early detection of the ICA in CS using intraoperative Doppler and visualize it at the level of the distal dural ring.

The presence of circular ingrowth of the ICA by the tumor cast doubt on attempts to separate them. Consequently, the sharp dissection of all involved vessels of the circle of Willis is preferred.

6.4 Veins

Venous anatomy in this region is extremely variable. They are always full-blooded and are at high risk of being damaged. The CS is a complex of venous channels. Due to the variability of the functional role of each vein, the excision of the tumor should be conducted with maintaining the integrity of the veins. They should be cut only if there is a confidence that the vein drains the tumor. Sylvian veins could be directly drained into the CS [15].

7. Surgical outcomes and prognosis

Sphenoid wing meningiomas are the group of tumors where the advantages of cranial base surgery over conventional transcranial surgery can be clearly demonstrated. The introduction of craniobasal approaches, which evolved from the fronto-temporal to the pterional and the fronto-temporo-orbito-zygomatic, and from the unilateral subfrontal to the fronto-lateral supraorbital, significantly reduces both the mortality and postoperative complications rate. Thus, in the 1970s postoperative mortality was up to 43% in some reports [37]. In contrast, nowadays less than 2% are reported [36]. The complication rate is dependent on involved structures and surgical approach but has markedly fallen over during the recent decades.

Analysis of the factors influencing the postoperative prognosis showed that histopathological characteristic of meningioma is one of the main determinants. Around 70% of meningiomas are benign (WHO grade I), while 28% are atypical (WHO grade II), and 2% are malignant (WHO grade III) [40]. Despite these well-known prognostic groups, meningiomas could have up to 15 different histologic subtypes. These characteristics are marked prognostic predictors and define the treatment strategy.

Anterolateral skull base and convexity meninges are derived from the neural crest, but the rest of the skull base has mesenchymal origin (paraxial mesoderm and dorsal mesoderm) [41]. This correlates with different histological subtypes of tumors and even WHO grades. Interestingly, the recent studies demonstrate the link between topography (meaning mesenchymal or neural crest origin) and the main somatic gene mutations [42].

The radicality of the removal is the next important prognostic factor. However, the introduction of radiosurgical treatment of the residual tumor of the skull base has significantly decreased the recurrence rate in the described group [42, 43].

8. Radiotherapy and radiosurgery

Surgical resection of MAC is the treatment of choice, but in some cases, surgery alone may not be radical due to the tumor invasion to the CS, ICA, and/or ON encasement. Subtotal resection with adjuvant postoperative radiotherapy may be preferable over complete resection.

High-dose fractionated radiotherapy and radiosurgery have been reported to achieve a tumor control rate between 93–97% and 91–98%, respectively [43]. Permanent complications after radiosurgery are rare and have been reported in 0–10.5% of patients. They mainly consist of delayed optic nerve neuropathy, trigeminal nerve dysfunction, cognitive deficits, and seizures [44]. Functional results after radiosurgery for meningiomas involving the CS have proved to be superior to those obtained after microsurgical resection. [45]

The growth pattern in progressive benign meningiomas after failed radiosurgery can be unusually aggressive. In the case of reoperation after radiotherapy, it is associated with a higher complication rate compared to primary procedures [46].

9. Conclusions

Despite the great variety of existing approaches, the pterional extradural is the most common "workhorse" for meningiomas of the anterior clinoidal process excision. If there is no clinoid process hyperostosis and cavernous sinus invasion, the fronto-lateral approach will be an option. Overall, total clinoidectomy is the key procedure for visualization of all important structures during an extradural way to the tumor. All the peculiarities should be taken into account to move safely and prevent the thermal and mechanical injury of neural and vascular structures. Radicality of excision is limited by the ICA encasement rate and character, the cavernous sinus invasion, and an anterior semicircle of Willis ingrowth. Preserving the integrity of perforating arteries and surrounding veins is the main key to preventing complications. Finally, the radicality of surgery will never exceed the value of the functional result of surgery and the patient's postoperative quality of life.

Conflict of interest

The authors declare no conflict of interest.

Author details

Oleksandr Voznyak and Nazarii Hryniv
Centre of Neurosurgery, Clinical Hospital "Feofaniya", Kyiv, Ukraine

*Address all correspondence to: drvoznyak@gmail.com

IntechOpen

References

[1] Al-Mefty O. Clinoidal meningiomas. Journal of Neurosurgery. 1990;**73**(6): 840-849. DOI: 10.3171/jns.1990.73. 6.0840

[2] Cushing H, Eisenhardt L. Meningiomas of the sphenoidal ridge. A. Those of the deep of clinoidal third. In: Cushing H, Eisenhardt L, editors. Meningiomas: Their Classification, Regional Behavior, Life History and Surgical End Results. Springfield, IL: Charles C Thomas; 1938. pp. 298-319

[3] Russell SM, Benjamin V. Medial sphenoid ridge meningiomas: Classification, microsurgical anatomy, operative nuances, and long-term surgical outcome in 35 consecutive patients. Neurosurgery. 2008;**62** (3, suppl 1):38-50. discussion 50

[4] Krisht A. Clinoidal meningiomas. In: DeMonte F, McDermott M, Al-Mefty O, editors. Al-Mefty's Meningiomas. 2nd ed. New York: Thieme Medical Publishers; 2011. pp. 297-306

[5] Bassiouni H, Asgari S, Sandalcioglu IE, Seifert V, Stolke D, Mar- quardt G. Anterior clinoidal meningiomas: functional outcome after microsurgical resection in a consecutive series of 106 patients: Clinical article. Journal of Neurosurgery. 2009;**111**(5): 1078-1090

[6] Güdük M, Özduman K, Pamir MN. Sphenoid Wing Meningiomas: Surgical Outcomes in a Series of 141 Cases and Proposal of a Scoring System Predicting Extent of Resection. World Neurosurgery. 2019;**125**:e48-e59. DOI: 10.1016/j.wneu.2018.12.175. Epub 2019 Jan 11

[7] Wang Z, Liang X, Yang Y, Gao B, Wang L, You W, et al. A new scoring system for predicting extent of resection in medial sphenoid wing meningiomas based on three-dimensional multimodality fusion imaging. Chinese Neurosurgical Journal. 2020;**6**(1):35. DOI: 10.1186/s41016-020-00214-0

[8] Chicoine M, Jost S. Surgical management of meningiomas of the sphenoidwing region: Operative approaches to medial and lateral sphenoid wing, spheno-orbital, and cavernous sinus meningiomas. In: Benham B, editor. Neurosurgical Operative Atlas: Neuro-oncology. 2nd ed. Rolling Meadows, IL: Thieme Medical Publishers and the American Association of Neurological Surgeons; 2007. pp. 161-169

[9] Forsting M, Jansen O. MR neuroimaging. In: Brain, Spine, Peripheral Nerves. Stuttgart, New York, Delhi, Rio de Janeiro: Thieme Publishers; 2017. p. 108. (582 pages). ISBN 978-3-13-202681-0, eISBN 978-3-13-202691-9

[10] Wanibuchi M, Friedmann AH, Fukushima T. Photo atlas of skull base dissection: Techniques and operative approaches. Annals of the Royal College of Surgeons of England. 2010;**92**(8):717. DOI: 10.1308/003588410X127718639374 03a

[11] Romani R, Elsharkawy A, Laakso A, Kangasniemi M, Hernesniemi J. Complications of anterior clinoidectomy through lateral supraorbital approach. World Neurosurgery. 2012;**77**(5-6):698-703. DOI: 10.1016/j.wneu.2011.08.014. Epub 2011 Nov 7

[12] Pamir MN, Belirgen M, Ozduman K, Kiliç T, Ozek M. Anterior clinoidal meningiomas: analysis of 43 consecutive surgically treated cases. Acta Neurochirurgica. 2008;**150**(7): 625-635. discussion 635-636

[13] Lee JH, Sade B, Park BJ. A surgical technique for the removal of clinoidal meningiomas. Neurosurgery. 2006;**59** (1 Suppl 1):ONS108-ONS114. discussion

ONS108-14. DOI: 10.1227/01.NEU. 0000220023.09021.03

[14] Lynch JC, Pereira CE, Gonçalves M, Zanon N. Extended pterional approach for medial sphenoid wing meningioma: A series of 47 patients. Journal of Neurological Surgery Part B: Skull Base. 2020;81(2):107-113. DOI: 10.1055/s-0039-1677728. Epub 2019 Feb 21

[15] Mitsuhashi Y, Hayasaki K, Kawakami T, Nagata T, Kaneshiro Y, Umaba R, et al. Dural venous system in the cavernous sinus: A literature review and embryological, functional, and endovascular clinical considerations. Neurologia Medico-Chirurgica (Tokyo). 2016;56(6):326-339. DOI: 10.2176/nmc. ra.2015-0346. Epub 2016 Apr 11

[16] Takahashi S, Sakuma I, Otani T, et al. Venous anatomy of the sphenoparietal sinus: Evaluation by MR imaging. Interventional Neuroradiology. 2007;13(Suppl 1):84-89. DOI: 10.1177/15910199070130S111

[17] Bonnal J, Thibaut A, Brotchi J, Born J. Invading meningiomas of the sphenoid ridge. Journal of Neurosurgery. 1980;53(5):587-599. Retrieved May 20, 2021, from https:// thejns.org/view/journals/j-neurosurg/ 53/5/article-p587.xml

[18] Simon M, Schramm J. Lateral and middle sphenoid wing meningiomas. In: DeMonte F, McDermott M, Al-Mefty O, editors. Al-Mefty's Meningiomas. 2nd ed. New York: Thieme Medical Publishers; 2011. pp. 297-306

[19] Vajkoczy P. Intradural versus extradural removal of the anterior clinoid process. World Neurosurgery. 2012;77(5-6):615-616. DOI: 10.1016/j. wneu.2011.10.026. Epub 2011 Nov 1

[20] Lehmberg J, Krieg SM, Meyer B. Anterior clinoidectomy. Acta Neurochirurgica. 2014;156(2):415-419; discussion 419. DOI: 10.1007/s00701-013-1960-1. Epub 2013 Dec 10

[21] Pieper DR, Al-Mefty O, Hanada Y, Buechner D. Hyperostosis associated with meningioma of the cranial base: secondary changes or tumor invasion. Neurosurgery. 1999;44(4):742-746. discussion 746-7. DOI: 10.1097/ 00006123-199904000-00028

[22] Bikmaz K, Mrak R, Al-Mefty O. Management of bone-invasive, hyperostotic sphenoid wing meningiomas. Journal of Neurosurgery. 2007;107(5):905-912. DOI: 10.3171/ JNS-07/11/0905

[23] Zamanipoor Najafabadi AH, Genders SW, van Furth WR. Visual outcomes endorse surgery of patients with spheno-orbital meningioma with minimal visual impairment or hyperostosis. Acta Neurochirurgica. 2021;163(1):73-82. DOI: 10.1007/ s00701-020-04554-9. Epub 2020 Sep 4

[24] Goyal N, Kakkar A, Sarkar C, Agrawal D. Does bony hyperostosis in intracranial meningioma signify tumor invasion? A radio-pathologic study. Neurology India. 2012;60(1):50-54. DOI: 10.4103/0028-3886.93589

[25] Corniola MV, Lemée JM, Schaller K, Meling TR. Lateral sphenoid wing meningiomas without bone invasion-still skull base surgery? Neurosurgical Review. 2020;43(6):1547-1553. DOI: 10.1007/s10143-019-01181-6. Epub 2019 Oct 29

[26] Salunke P, Sahoo SK, Singh A, Yagnick N. Arteries paving the way for centrifugal excision of anterior clinoidal meningioma. World Neurosurgery. 2018;117:65. DOI: 10.1016/j.wneu. 2018.06.013. Epub 2018 Jun 12

[27] Salunke P, Singh A, Kamble R, Ahuja C. Vascular involvement in anterior clinoidal meningiomas: Biting the 'artery' that feeds. Clinical Neurology and Neurosurgery. 2019 Sep;184:105413. DOI: 10.1016/j. clineuro.2019.105413. Epub 2019 Jul 6

[28] Whittle IR, Smith C, Navoo P, Collie D. Meningiomas. Lancet. 2004;**363**(9420):1535-1543. DOI: 10.1016/S0140-6736(04)16153-9

[29] Toh CH, Castillo M, Wong AM, Wei KC, Wong HF, Ng SH, et al. Differentiation between classic and atypical meningiomas with use of diffusion tensor imaging. AJNR. American Journal of Neuroradiology. 2008;**29**(9):1630-1635. DOI: 10.3174/ajnr.A1170. Epub 2008 Jun 26

[30] Champagne PO, Lemoine E, Bojanowski MW. Surgical management of giant sphenoid wing meningiomas encasing major cerebral arteries. Neurosurgical Focus. 2018;**44**(4):E12. DOI: 10.3171/2018.1.FOCUS17718 PMID: 29606042

[31] Honig S, Trantakis C, Frerich B, Sterker I, Kortmann RD, Meixensberger J. Meningiomas involving the sphenoid wing outcome after microsurgical treatment--a clinical review of 73 cases. Central European Neurosurgery. 2010;**71**(4):189-198. DOI: 10.1055/s-0030-1261945

[32] Attia M, Umansky F, Paldor I, Dotan S, Shoshan Y, Spektor S. Giant anterior clinoidal meningiomas: surgical technique and outcomes. Journal of Neurosurgery. 2012;**117**(4):654-665. DOI: 10.3171/2012.7.JNS111675

[33] Wiedemayer H, Sandalcioglu IE, Wiedemayer H, Stolke D. The supraorbital keyhole approach via an eyebrow incision for resection of tumors around the sella and the anterior skull base. Minimally Invasive Neurosurgery. 2004;**47**(4):221-225. DOI: 10.1055/s-2004-818526

[34] Borghei-Razavi H, Truong HQ, Fernandes-Cabral DT, Celtikci E, Chabot JD, Stefko ST, et al. Minimally invasive approaches for anterior skull base meningiomas: Supraorbital eyebrow, endoscopic endonasal, or a combination of both? anatomic study, limitations, and surgical application. World Neurosurgery. 2018;**112**:e666-e674. DOI: 10.1016/j.wneu.2018.01.119. Epub 2018 Feb 19

[35] Dossani RH, Kalakoti P, Guthikonda B. Supraorbital approach for resection of clinoidal meningioma. World Neurosurgery. 2018;**109**:295. DOI: 10.1016/j.wneu.2017.10.019. Epub 2017 Oct 13

[36] Sughrue ME, Rutkowski MJ, Chen CJ, Shangari G, Kane AJ, Parsa AT, et al. Modern surgical outcomes following surgery for sphenoid wing meningiomas. Journal of Neurosurgery. 2013;**119**(1):86-93. DOI: 10.3171/2012.12.JNS11539. Epub 2013 Feb 22

[37] Corell A, Thurin E, Skoglund T, Farahmand D, Henriksson R, Rydenhag B, et al. Neurosurgical treatment and outcome patterns of meningioma in Sweden: A nationwide registry-based study. Acta Neurochirurgica. 2019;**161**(2):333-341. DOI: 10.1007/s00701-019-03799-3. Epub 2019 Jan 24

[38] Sakata K, Suematsu K, Takeshige N, Nagata Y, Orito K, Miyagi N, et al. Novel method of intraoperative ocular movement monitoring using a piezoelectric device: experimental study of ocular motor nerve activating piezoelectric potentials (OMNAPP) and clinical application for skull base surgeries. Neurosurgical Review. 2020;**43**(1):185-193. DOI: 10.1007/s10143-018-1028-z. Epub 2018 Sep 12

[39] Schlake HP, Goldbrunner R, Siebert M, Behr R, Roosen K. Intra-Operative electromyographic monitoring of extra-ocular motor nerves (Nn. III, VI) in skull base surgery. Acta Neurochirurgica. 2001;**143**(3):251-261. DOI: 10.1007/s007010170105

[40] Louis DN, Perry A, Reifenberger G, von Deimling A, Figarella-Branger D,

Cavenee WK, et al. The 2016 World Health Organization classification of tumors of the central nervous system: A summary. Acta Neuropathologica. 2016 Jun;**131**(6):803-820. DOI: 10.1007/s00401-016-1545-1. Epub 2016 May 9

[41] Del Maestro R. Al-Mefty's Meningiomas. Second Edition. 2011. Edited by Franco DeMonte, Michael W. McDermott, Ossama Al-Mefty. Published by Thieme Medical Publishers, Inc. 432pages. C$210 approx. Canadian Journal of Neurological Sciences / Journal Canadien Des Sciences Neurologiques. 2013;**40**(1):131-132. DOI: 10.1017/S0317167100017455

[42] Jensen RL, Minshew L, Shrieve AF, Hu N, Shrieve DC. Stereotactic radiosurgery and radiotherapy for meningiomas: Biomarker predictors of patient outcome and response to therapy. Journal of Radiosurgery & SBRT. 2012;**2**(1):41-50

[43] Starke RM, Przybylowski CJ, Sugoto M, Fezeu F, Awad AJ, Ding D, et al. Gamma Knife radiosurgery of large skull base meningiomas. Journal of Neurosurgery JNS. 2015;**122**(2):363-372. Retrieved Jul 21, 2021, from: https://thejns.org/view/journals/j-neurosurg/122/2/article-p363.xml

[44] Akyoldaş G, Hergünsel ÖB, Yılmaz M, Şengöz M, Peker S. Gamma knife radiosurgery for anterior clinoid process meningiomas: A series of 61 consecutive patients. World Neurosurgery. 2020;**133**:e529-e534. DOI: 10.1016/j.wneu.2019.09.089. Epub 2019 Sep 25

[45] Lippitz BE, Bartek J Jr, Mathiesen T, Förander P. Ten-year follow-up after Gamma Knife radiosurgery of meningioma and review of the literature. Acta Neurochirurgica. 2020;**162**(9):2183-2196. DOI: 10.1007/s00701-020-04350-5. Epub 2020 Jun 26

[46] Cohen-Inbar O, Tata A, Moosa S, Lee CC, Sheehan JP. Stereotactic radiosurgery in the treatment of parasellar meningiomas: Long-term volumetric evaluation. Journal of Neurosurgery. 2018;**128**(2):362-372. DOI: 10.3171/2016.11.JNS161402. Epub 2017 Mar 24

Section 4

Pituitary Adenomas

Chapter 5

Pituitary Adenomas: Classification, Clinical Evaluation and Management

Bilal Ibrahim, Mauricio Mandel, Assad Ali, Edinson Najera, Michal Obrzut, Badih Adada and Hamid Borghei-Razavi

Abstract

Pituitary adenomas are one of the most common brain tumors. They represent approximately 18% of all intracranial, and around 95% of sellar neoplasms. In recent years, our understanding of the pathophysiology and the behavior of these lesions has led to better control and higher curative rates. The treatment decision is largely dependent on type of the adenoma, clinical presentation, and the size of the lesion. In addition, incidental pituitary lesions add uncertainty in the decision-making process, especially for pituitary adenomas that can be medically managed. When surgery is indicated, the endoscopic endonasal transsphenoidal approach is the technique of choice, but open standard craniotomy approaches can also be the option in selected cases. The following chapter will review the classification, clinical presentation, pathophysiology, diagnostic work-up, selection of surgical approach, and treatment complications in pituitary adenomas.

Keywords: functional pituitary adenomas, non-functional pituitary adenomas, sellar tumor, endoscopic endonasal surgery, prolactinoma, acromegaly, Cushing's disease

1. Introduction

Pituitary adenomas (PA) are benign tumors which account for being the second most common intracranial tumors after meningiomas [1]. The incidence of PA is 4.36 per 100,000 and can affect all age groups [1]. However, PA is uncommon in the 1st decade of life with a prevalence of 1–10% when compared to all brain tumors in that age group [2]. The overall chance of developing a pituitary adenoma increases with age, and the non-secretory type is most common after 40 years old [2, 3]. Presentation is highly dependent on the whether the tumor is capable to disrupt hormone homeostasis. Secretory adenomas, also called "functional" adenomas, tend to present early in the clinical course of disease. Conversely, non-secreting adenomas, also called non-functional" adenomas, typically present after reaching a critical size, leading to compression of surrounding neuronal and/or vascular structures.

The first step in the management of a patient with a pituitary adenoma is to distinguish the lesion between a secreting and a non-secreting one. The secreting-type subclassification is based on the specific hormone release by the tumor. Despite advancements in pharmacologic and radiotherapeutic management, surgery is still considered the main modality of treatment for most pituitary adenomas.

2. Applied anatomy and general information

The pituitary gland is located in the hypophyseal fossa, which is a depression in body of the sphenoid bone located in the middle cranial fossa. Anteriorly, this space is limited by the tuberculum sellae, posteriorly by the dorsum sellae, laterally by the medial wall of the cavernous sinus on each side which extends from the anterior clinoid process and superior orbital fissure anteriorly to the posterior clinoid process posteriorly (**Figure 1A**). The chiasmatic sulcus is a shallow depression running between tuberculum sellae and the limbus sphenoidale where the optic chiasm spans between two optic nerves. The anterior tip of the chiasmatic sulcus, or limbus sphenoidale, is the limit between the anterior and middle cranial fossae. The pituitary gland is an intradural extra-arachnoidal structure with an ovoid shape composed of two lobes: a larger anterior lobe and a smaller posterior one. The pituitary stalk (aka the infundibulum) provides the pathway for ascending neural connections arising from superior surface of the posterior lobe to the hypothalamus.

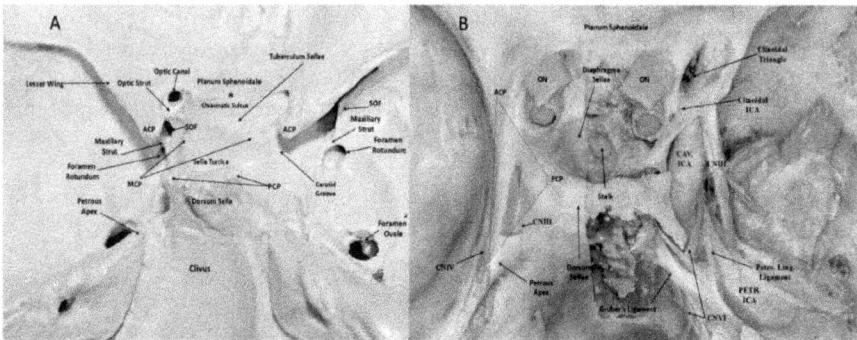

Figure 1.
Intracranial view showing sellar and parasellar areas anatomy. A: Superior view of cranial base. Hypophyseal fossa, or sellae turcica, bounded anteriorly by tuberculum sellae, posteriorly by the dorsum sellae, laterally by the medial wall of the cavernous sinus on each side which extends form anterior clinoid process and superior orbital fissure (SOF) anteriorly to posterior clinoid process posteriorly. Anterior tip of chiasmatic sulcus called limbus sphenoidale (marked by asterisk) which is the junction between anterior and middle cranial fossa. Anterior optic strut separates optic canal superomedially from SOF inferolatearlly and maxillary strut separates SOF from foramen rotundum. Middle clinoid process (MCP), which present in 50% of population, is a projection from lateral margin of sellae turcica. It corresponds transsphenoidally to medial opticocarotid recess. B: Superior view showing the roof hypophyseal fossa and cavernous sinus. Diaphragm sellae roof the superior surface of pituitary gland with the exception of a small opening that allows the stalk to pass from the gland to the hypothalamus. It is continuous with the dura covering the planum sphenoidale anteriorly and the dorsum sellae and clivus posteriorly. The roof of cavernous sinus formed by the oculomotor triangle (blue highlighted triangle) and clinoidal triangle. Oculomotor nerve (CNIII) enter the cavernous sinus at the middle of oculomotor triangle. The roof of left cavernous sinus is opened to show the contents of the cavernous sinus. Only the ICA and abducens nerve (CN VI) are running inside the sinus. CNIII, trochlear (CNIV), ophthalmic, and maxillary nerve are running in the lateral wall of cavernous sinus. CN VI enters the cavernous sinus by passing under Gruber's ligament (aka petrosphenoidal ligament) which spans from the petrous apex to the posterior clinoid process and form the roof of Dorello's canal. In this specimen, Gruber's ligament is duplicated. ACP, anterior clinoid process; CAV. ICA, cavernous segment of ICA; MCP, middle clinoid process; PCP, posterior clinoid process; ON, optic nerve; PETR. ICA, petrous segment of ICA.

Due to the lack of a robust blood-brain barrier, the pituitary gland exhibits intense enhancement on contrasted magnetic resonance imaging (MRI). The larger anterior pituitary gland is composed of 3 parts:

1. Pars distalis (anterior): the largest of the 3 parts, responsible for the bulk of hormone production.

2. Pars tuberalis: an upward extension of glandular cell sheaths that connects the pars distalis to the pituitary stalk.

3. Pars intermedia: epithelial cells that sheath and separate the pars distalis from the pars tuberalis.

Five types of endocrine cells are contained inside the anterior lobe that secrete 6 different hormones (**Table 1**). The secretion of hormones is under either stimulatory control from hypothalamus or inhibitory control through feed-back mechanisms. Prolactin is the only pituitary hormone that is under inhibitory control from hypothalamus by prolactin releasing inhibitory factor, mainly dopamine.

The roof of the sellae is formed by a structure known as the diaphragm sellae, which covers the entire superior surface of pituitary gland with the exception of a small opening that allows the stalk to pass from the gland to the hypothalamus. It is formed by a dual layer of dura that is continuous with the dura covering the planum sphenoidale anteriorly and the dorsum sellae and clivus posteriorly (**Figure 1B**).

Anterior lobe					
Pituitary cell	**Hormone produced**	**Control**	**Staining**	**Target organ**	**Effects**
Corticotrophs	ACTH	⊕CRH	Basophile	Adrenal gland	Cortisol secretion
Thyrotrophs	TSH	⊕TRH	Basophile	Thyroid gland	T3 & T4 secretion
Gonadotrophs	LH, FSH	⊕GnRH	Basophile	Gonads	♂: Testosterone ♀: Estradiol
Somatotrophs	GH	⊕GHRH ⊖Somatostatin	Acidophile	Epiphyses of long bones Liver	Bones: Chondrocyte proliferation Liver: IGF-1 release
Lactotrophs	PRL*	⊖PIF	Acidophile	Mammillary gland	Lactation
Posterior lobe					
Hormone produced		**Target organ**		**Effects**	
Antidiuretic hormone (ADH)		Kidneys		Fluid retention, vasoconstriction	
Oxytocin		Uterine smooth muscle Mammary gland		Uterine contraction Milk ejection into lactation ducts	

Prolactin is the only hormone that is under direct inhibition from hypothalamus.
ACTH, adrenocorticotropic hormone; FSH, follicle-stimulating hormone; GH, growth hormone; GHRH, growth hormone releasing hormone; LH, luteinizing hormone; PRL, prolactin; TSH, thyroid-stimulating hormone.

Table 1.
Pituitary glandular cell types and function.

Two layers of dura cover the sellar anterior wall and the floor, namely: the inner (meningeal) layer, and the outer (periosteal) layer. These dural layers run adherent to each other on the anterior and floor of the hypophyseal fossa. Laterally, these 2 dural layers split, as the outer layer continues laterally and form the anterior wall of the cavernous sinus, and the inner layer adheres to lateral wall of pituitary gland to form the medial wall of cavernous sinus (**Figure 2**). Inferior and superior inter-cavernous sinuses are venous channels that connect the bilateral cavernous sinuses to each other. These venous channels run in the space between the two dural layers in superior and inferior aspects of the hypophyseal fossa (**Figure 2**). In extended transsphenoidal approaches, it is important to coagulate those venous channels before dural opening to avoid significant venous bleeding.

The floor of the sellae forms the posterior wall of sphenoidal sinus, which offers a shortcut in approaching the sellar region. The sphenoidal sinus can be classified based on the degree of pneumatization: conchal, presellar, and sellar. The sellar type is the most common and it is found in 80% of population, representing of a fully pneumatized sphenoid sinus. The conchal type is present in 3% of the population, and it represents a non-pneumatized form. It is common to see this type in the pediatric age population as aeration begins at 10 months of age and rapidly progresses between ages 3 and 6 years—eventually achieving final pneumatization around the 3rd decade of life. The presellar type is an intermediate classification between the conchal and sellar types in which partial pneumatization is observed.

During the endonasal transsphenoidal approach to the sellar and suprasellar regions important structures can be identified as bony prominences on the posterior wall of sphenoidal sinus depending on the degree of aeration. These include the cavernous carotid artery prominences, optic nerves prominences, pituitary gland prominence, and paraclival carotids segments prominences. The lateral optic

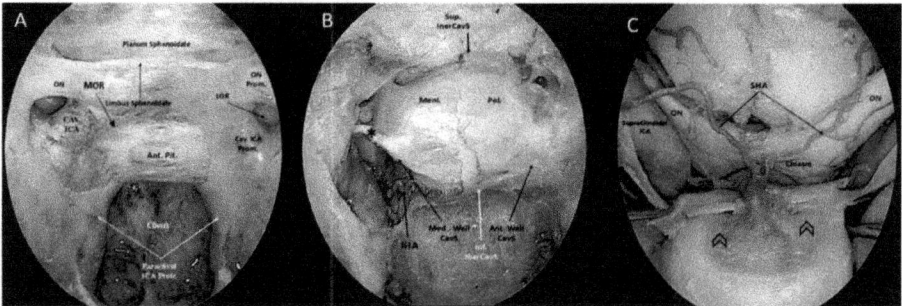

Figure 2.
Transsphenoidal endoscopic stepwise dissection of sellar floor. (A) Sellar floor bone over the right side anterior wall of cavernous sinus and pituitary gland has been removed and kept intact on the left side. Important landmarks can be appreciated on the sellar floor. Optic nerve, cavernous and paraclival ICA segments prominences can be seen. Lateral opticocarotid recess (LOR) seen superolateral to carotid prominence and inferior to optic nerve prominence (ON Prom.), and it corresponds to optic strut. Limbus sphenoidale spans between optic chiasm/chiasmatic sulcus and planum sphenoidale. (B) Bone over sellar floor removed completely. Periosteal layer of dura (PoL) has been peeled from the meningeal layer (MenL) on the right half of the gland and kept on the left. The anterior wall of cavernous sinus formed by PoL after separating form MenL on the lateral aspect of the pituitary gland and MenL remains stuck to the gland forming the medial wall of cavernous sinus. Note the ligament (marked by "*") that anchor the medial wall of cavernous sinus. Also, those 2 layers separate at superior and inferior aspects of pituitary gland to form superior intercavernous sinus (Sup. InterCavS.) and inferior intercavernous sinus (Inf. InterCavS.), respectively, which are venous channels connecting the bilateral cavernous sinuses. Inferior hypophyseal artery (IHA) is a branch from meningohypophyseal trunk in majority of cases and supply the pituitary gland with blood. (C) Dura over sellae and suprasellar area has been removed to show the superior hypophyseal artery (SHA) which is a direct branch from supraclinoidal segment of ICA to supply the stalk and gland in addition to optic chiasm and nerves. The arrow heads pointing to diaphragma sellae. Note the opening in the diaphragm through which the stalk ascends from the gland to hypothalamus.

carotid recess is a depression seen between internal carotid artery (ICA) and the optic nerve prominences. This structure correlates with the optic strut/anterior clinoid process when viewed transcranially (**Figure 2**).

2.1 Blood supply of pituitary gland

The pituitary gland receives its blood supply from bilateral superior and inferior hypophyseal arteries. Superior hypophyseal artery (SHA) is a direct branch from the supraclinoidal segment of the ICA. In addition to supplying the pituitary gland and stalk, the SHA also supplies the optic nerve and chiasm. The inferior hypophyseal artery (IHA) branches from the cavernous segment of the ICA, but can also branch from the meningohypophyseal trunk. The IHA supplies the pituitary gland and to some extent the stalk (**Figure 2**). Truong et al. [4] found that the bilateral coagulation of IHA has minimal effect on adenohypophysis and neurohypophysis functions due to presence of rich intraarterial anastomosis between SHAs. However, injury to SHA branches supplying the visual apparatus may result in visual field defects or vision loss due to paucity of anastomosis in the optic nerves or chiasm.

3. Classification of pituitary adenomas

Multiple classification systems have been adopted to classify pituitary adenomas. They can be classified either based on functioning status (i.e. secretory and non-secretory) or on the size of the adenoma (i.e. >1 cm in diameter macroadenoma, <1 cm diameter microadenoma). Other classification systems include pathological findings under light microscopy with hematoxylin and eosin stains (basophilic, acidophilic, or chromophobic), or growth characteristics found on imaging studies (e.g. modified Hardy's classification for suprasellar extension and Knosp classification for parasellar/cavernous sinus extension).

The functional classification is the most widely used. It classifies pituitary adenomas on the hormone secretion status and the resultant endocrinologic manifestation. Functioning adenomas may secrete PRL, GH, ACTH, TSH, or FSH/LH, and patients usually present with endocrinologic manifestations of endogenous effect of the hyper-secreted hormone. Non-functioning adenomas usually present with mass effect on surrounding neuronal or vascular structures or with pituitary dysfunction due to compression on normal glandular tissue.

4. Clinical presentation

Pituitary adenomas may present with multiple different manifestations. These include: hormonal hypersecretory signs and symptoms, pituitary dysfunction, mass effect on surrounding neuronal structures, or may present acutely with headache and altered mental status due to pituitary apoplexy. However, asymptomatic pituitary adenomas discovered incidentally on brain MRI are not uncommon. It was found that 10% of general adult population may have asymptomatic pituitary adenoma (pituitary incidentalomas) [5].

4.1 Hormonal manifestations

One of the most common clinical presentation of pituitary adenomas is hormonal disturbances. Hypersecretion of one of the pituitary hormones will result in distinctive clinical syndrome that is related to endogenous effect of the hormone (**Table 2**).

Adenoma type	Incidence[*]	Hormone in excess	Clinical manifestation
Prolactinoma	40–57%	PRL	Male: decrease libido, impotence. Female: amenorrhea-galactorrhea syndrome Either sex: infertility, osteoporosis, headache, visual changes
GH cell (somatotroph) adenoma	11%	GH	Acromegaly
Corticotroph adenoma	2%	ACTH	Cushing's disease
Thyrotroph adenoma	Rare	TSH	Hyperthyroidism
Gonadotroph adenoma	Rare	LH, FSH	Mostly present as non-secretory adenoma; rarely may cause menstrual abnormalities, ovarian hyperstimulation syndrome, and in males may cause testicular enlargement, hypogonadism

Incidence of all pituitary adenomas [41].

Table 2.
Functional pituitary adenomas clinical presentation.

4.2 Pituitary dysfunction

Pituitary dysfunction is generally caused by the adenoma compression over normal secretory glandular tissue or the pituitary stalk. Usually, significant tumor growth (size >1 cm) and pituitary compression is needed to cause pituitary dysfunction. GH is the first hormone to be affected, followed by LH and FSH, then TSH and lastly ACTH. Single hormonal dysfunction due to pituitary compression is extremely rare. Pituitary stalk compression may result in hyperprolactinemia due to the loss of inhibitory control from hypothalamus which manifest as a moderate elevation in prolactin level (usually <150 μg/l).

4.3 Mass effect

Pituitary macroadenomas may extend to the suprasellar region causing compression to the optic nerves and chiasm. Visual impairment is seen in about 40–60% of patients upon presentation and the classical presentation is bitemporal hemianopsia. In addition, suprasellar mass growth may result in hypothalamic compression with subsequent disturbances in eating, emotion or sleep pattern. Rarely, 3rd ventricle extension may result in obstructive hydrocephalus. Parasellar extension into cavernous sinus is usually asymptomatic, however, oculomotor, abducens and trigeminal nerves compressive symptoms may occur. Additional parasellar extension may compress the mesial temporal lobe which can result in seizures.

4.4 Pituitary apoplexy

Pituitary apoplexy is defined as sudden onset of intense headache associated with visual field defects, ophthalmoplegia, and/or altered mental status [6]. Pituitary apoplexy is clinically observed in 1–7% of pituitary adenomas [6, 7]. The accepted pathophysiology is tumor outgrowth of the vascular blood supply resulting in hemorrhagic infarction of the tumor mass [8]. Headache is the most common symptom which is usually felt over frontal or retro-orbital areas. However, visual field defects, cranial nerves palsy, and meningeal irritation signs and symptoms are not uncommon. Approximately 80% of patients have anterior pituitary hormonal dysfunction with ACTH deficiency being the most critical one.

There is evidence suggesting that the risk of pituitary apoplexy is higher in functional pituitary adenomas (e.g. GH-secreting adenomas and prolactinomas). However, there is contradicting data demonstrating a higher risk in non-functional ones [7]. Multiple risk factors for pituitary apoplexy have been identified including; sudden changes in blood pressure, (e.g. major surgeries), coagulative disorders and anticoagulation usage, radiotherapy, estrogen-based oral contraceptive pills, and head trauma [6, 7, 9].

5. Prolactinoma

Prolactinoma is the most common type in secretary pituitary adenoma with an incidence of 50% of all pituitary adenomas. It is typically commonly seen in women aged 20–50 years old. As stated previously, prolactin is under continuous inhibition from dopamine, a PIF, secreted from hypothalamus through the pituitary stalk. Stalk dysfunction, either by compression or hypothalamic lesion, will result in loss of prolactin inhibition with subsequent prolactin elevation. Prolactinomas arise from monoclonal expansion of pituitary lactotrophs, however, 5–10% of prolactinomas can co-secrete GH resulting in superimposed gigantism/acromegaly [10]. As the disruption of hormone homeostasis causes subtle symptoms in some prolactinoma patients, it is the most likely tumor to become large enough to cause clinical manifestations of mass effect compared to other secreting tumors.

5.1 Signs and symptoms

Hyperprolactinemia symptoms in males include decreased libido, sexual dysfunction and oligozoospermia (due to secondary hypogonadism). In perimenopause females, amenorrhea-galactorrhea syndrome is usually seen, which is a triad of galactorrhea, amenorrhea and infertility. In children and adolescents, growth arrest, pubertal delay and primary amenorrhea are frequently seen. Symptoms may also be due to mass effect which may cause headache, vision field deficits, cranial nerve palsy, seizure, and hydrocephalus.

Head trauma
Convulsions
Medication (antipsychotics, antiemetics, verapamil)
Chest wall stimulation, strenuous exercises, heavy meals.
Craniopharyngioma, granulomatous disease of the hypothalamus, acromegaly
Primary hypothyroidism
Pregnancy and breast feeding

Table 3.
Differential diagnosis of hyperprolactinemia.

5.2 Evaluation

Diagnosis of prolactinoma requires both: radiological evidence of adenoma and sustained hyperprolactinemia. Normal PRL levels in women are <25 µg/l and in men are <20 µg/l. Single random measurement of PRL at any time of the day is adequate for evaluation of hyperprolactinemia. The differential diagnosis of hyperprolactinemia is wide (**Table 3**), but PRL level is seldom >100 µg/l in these conditions. Pituitary stalk compression (Stalk Effect) can also cause hyperprolactinemia (e.g. PRL level up to 150 µg/l) [11, 12].

In PRL-secreting adenomas, PRL level usually correlates with tumor size as levels above 250 µg/l are commonly seen in macroadenomas [12]. In the setting of low PRL level in patients with clinical presentation strongly suggestive of a prolactinoma, "hook effect" should be suspected. Hook effect occurs due to the impairment of immune-complex formation in the presence of high levels of PRL. To overcome this phenomenon, serial dilution of the sample with repetition of the immunoassay is needed.

After ruling-out other causes of hyperprolactinemia, diagnosis confirmation of prolactinoma is made by gadolinium-enhanced brain MRI.

5.3 Management

Management of prolactinomas depends on several factors: tumor size, patient symptoms and preferences, and PRL level. All patients with macroadenoma require treatment, however, mildly symptomatic microadenoma patients (e.g. premenopausal woman with normal menstrual cycles and galactorrhea, or postmenopausal woman with tolerable galactorrhea) can be followed-up with serial PRL level measurement and brain MRI. Since only 5–10% of microadenomas will enlarge in size [13], management of microadenomas should not be based on size control alone. Prolactinomas respond very well to medical therapy, and dopamine agonists are the first line of management (e.g. bromocriptine or cabergoline) (**Table 4**).

Bromocriptine is a non-selective dopamine receptor agonist. It is the first line of management for microadenoma patients seeking fertility restoration and it is effective in 90% of patients and PRL level normalization can be achieved in 82% of patients [14]. If pregnancy has been achieved, bromocriptine can be stopped safely without a risk of abortion or congenital malformation. In child-bearing age women

Dopamine agonist	Bromocriptine	Cabergoline
Mode of action	Ergot-derivate D1 and D2 receptors agonist	Non-ergot-derivate Selective D2 agonist
starting dosage	1.25 mg/day	0.5 mg/week
Desired dosage	1.25 mg increment weekly until 2.5 mg × 3/day is reached	0.5 mg increment monthly until maximum dose of 3 mg/week is reached
Side effects	Gastrointestinal (GI) upset, postural hypotension, peripheral vasodilation, mood disturbances	GI upset, headache, dizziness, hypotension, cardiac valve fibrosis (mitral valve most commonly affected)
Response rate [14]	Microadenoma: normalize PRL in 82%, gonadal function restoration in 90% Macroadenoma: 80% will reduce in size	Microadenoma: 70% effective in bromocriptine resistant patients with fewer side effects rate Macroadenoma: higher tumor size control compared to bromocriptine

Table 4.
Bromocriptine and cabergoline specifications.

with microadenomas, risk of microadenoma progression is low and prolactin level monitoring is not necessary [15].

Macroadenomas always need management. Bromocriptine should be the drug of choice for patients who need fertility restoration. Pregnant women with macroadenoma without extrasellar extension can be followed similarly as microadenoma patients. However, if the suprasellar extension was detected before pregnancy, tumor debulking is advisable as the risk of macroadenoma growth during pregnancy is up to 35% [15, 16]. In these patients, it is also prudent to have a visual field assessment every 3 months till delivery.

Surgical management of prolactinoma is indicated in patients who are non-responders to dopaminergic therapy, with intolerable adverse effects from medical therapy (e.g. bromocriptine), CSF fistulas under DA, cystic tumors with intramural hemorrhage, or progressive neurological deficits [11, 17]. Stable visual field defect is not considered an indication for surgery as most patients will have tumor shrinkage on medical therapy with improvement on visual symptoms.

When to consider a prolactinoma as being medication resistant?

1. Failure to normalize serum prolactin levels after having received a daily dose of 15 mg of Bromocriptine for 3 months (25% of patients).

2. Failure to normalize serum prolactin levels after having received a weekly dose of 1.5–3.0 mg of Cabergoline for 3 months (10–15% of patients).

Seventy-percent of bromocriptine resistant patients will respond on cabergoline. Around 10–16% of prolactinoma patients will need surgical management [11]. Most patients will have a reduction of PRL levels 2–3 weeks after dopamine agonist initiation, which generally precedes the tumor size reduction. Periodic PRL measurements and pituitary MRI every 6–12 months is advised. After 2 years of continuous therapy, if prolactin levels have been normalized and >50% reduction of tumor size has been achieved, medication dose can be reduced. Typically, a low-dose of dopamine agonist after 2 years of tumor control will usually keep prolactin within normal range and prevent tumor recurrence [18].

6. Acromegaly and gigantism

Acromegaly is a rare disorder resulting from exposure to high levels of GH which is associated with significant morbidity and mortality. The most common cause of acromegaly is pituitary adenomas which may be either pure-GH secreting adenoma (60%) or mixed cell adenoma. In children before epiphyseal plate closure, GH secreting adenoma results in gigantism. It has an annual prevalence of 4 new cases per million inhabitants, with male and female being equally affected [19]. Other rare causes of acromegaly include growth hormone releasing hormone (GHRH) secretion from hypothalamus (e.g. hamartoma or glioma) or ectopic GHRH secreting tumors (e.g. primary bronchial carcinoid or pancreatic cancers).

6.1 Clinical presentation

The majority of acromegaly cases are due to GH-secreting pituitary adenomas. Similar to other subtypes of pituitary adenomas, GH-secreting adenomas may present with mass effect symptoms and/or with signs and symptoms of the endogenous effect of the over secreted hormone (i.e. GH).

Acromegaly dysmorphic features include enlarged hands and feet, facial bone enlargement that results in frontal bossing, prognathism, maxillary widening with the resultant of teeth separation and jaw malocclusion. The pathophysiology of bone changes is due to GH/IGF-1 effects on the periosteum of bones that results in new bone formation and bone remodeling. In the extremities, these effects will result in osteophyte formation over the digits with cartilage hypertrophy. Radiological hand findings include joint spaces widening, enthesopathy, diaphysis broadening and soft tissue hypertrophy. Due to these changes, two-thirds of patients will have degenerative arthropathy with large joints more commonly affected. In fact, arthropathy is the most common symptom referred by patients with acromegaly on presentation and the leading cause of morbidity. The axial skeleton can be affected by the same mechanism resulting in excessive kyphotic angulation of the thoracic spine with a compensatory hyperlordotic angulation of lumber vertebrae. These factors contribute to the fact that approximately half of these patients have low back pain. Neurogenic claudication is not uncommon due to ligamentum flavum hypertrophy with the resultant spinal canal stenosis. Patients with pure somatotroph pituitary adenoma usually have normal bone mineral density, however, acromegaly patients showed a higher incidence of vertebral compression fractures with high IGF-1 being a significant risk factor [20].

Growth Hormone and insulin like growth factor 1 can also affect visceral organs. Up to 50% of acromegaly patients have hypertension [21, 22]. The underlying cause is multifactorial. Endothelial dysfunction can be caused by GH-induced hyper-reactivity of the sympathetic nervous system [23]. In addition, high levels of GH/IGF-1 increase sodium reabsorption in renal distal tubules which results in chronic water retention/hypervolemia and increased plasma volume (up to 40%) when compared with normal individuals. Another important cause is chronic-sleep-apnea-induced hypertension as 80% of acromegaly patients have obstructive-sleep apnea induced by soft tissue hypertrophy. In addition, hypertrophic cardiomyopathy is commonly found in long standing acromegaly with diastolic dysfunction being the most common cardiac manifestation. Moreover, premature ventricular contractions can be detected in up to 50% of patients. The most common cause of mortality in acromegaly patients is due to cardiac arrhythmias or dysfunction [19].

Acromegaly has deleterious effects on both the upper and lower respiratory systems. Costal bone and subsequently chest wall changes (e.g. barrel chest) are common. Intercostal muscles also are affected by segmental degenerative fibrotic changes resulting weak inspiratory and expiratory efforts [24]. In the upper respiratory tract, acromegaly patients develop macroglossia, narrowing of pharyngeal airway space and thickening of vocal cords. These changes contribute largely to the pathogenesis of obstructive sleep apnea. One third of acromegalic patients with sleep apnea have neurogenic causes due to the effect of GH/IGF-1 on the respiratory center in the brain stem. Total lung capacity is increased in the majority of acromegalic patients due to increased alveolar volume. Narrowing of bronchi and bronchioles lead to obstructive patterns found in approximately 30% of patients, but they rarely have hypoxia due to the absence of ventilation-perfusion mismatch.

In the intestine, increased GH results in an incidence of colon polyps and cancer. Delhougne et al. [25] found in a prospective study that 45% of acromegalic patients had colonic polyps, 24% of them were of the adenomatous type. IGF-1 is unique in that it induces cellular growth and proliferation while also possessing an anti-apoptogenic effect. In 2010, The British Society of Gastroenterology (BSG) and the Association of Coloproctology for Great Britain and Ireland (ACPGBI) advised to start screening of acromegaly patients at the age of 40 with colonoscopy, 10 years earlier than the general population. Patients who were found to have adenoma at first screening *or* an increased serum IGF1 level above the maximum of the age-corrected normal range needed to be screened every 3 years. Patients with normal colonoscopy or non-adenomatous polyp, or normal growth hormone/IGF1 level, should be screened every 5–10 years [26].

6.2 Evaluation

Due to its pulsatile nature of secretion, random GH measurement is not preferred. Clinical diagnosis starts by observing the typical manifestations of GH hypersecretion (**Figure 3**). Once it is suspected, early morning GH level and IGF-1 level are measured. It is highly advised to use sex and age adjusted levels of IGF-1 as variations in the levels may result in false negative results. The gold standard test for acromegaly diagnosis confirmation is oral-glucose tolerance test (OGTT).

All patients with confirmed acromegaly should be screened for associated comorbidities which include hypertension, diabetes, cardiomyopathy and ECG, sleep apnea, and colonoscopy if the age above >40 years old. Patients who have acromegaly related comorbidities have two-fold increase in mortality [24]. While clinical manifestation is extremely indicative of the type of pituitary adenoma—lab values for other pituitary hormones are important screening factors for mixed adenomas (e.g. PRL co-secretion is found in 30% of patients). Standard visual field assessment should be offered to all patients who have macroadenomas abutting the visual apparatus on imaging studies.

Pituitary MRI is needed for evaluation of acromegaly of pituitary source. Because of its insidious onset, GH secreting pituitary adenomas present around 4–7 years after onset. At the time of diagnosis, around 75% of acromegaly patients have macroadenoma on MRI. It is important to note the extent of invasion to suprasellar and cavernous sinus compartments (**Figure 4**).

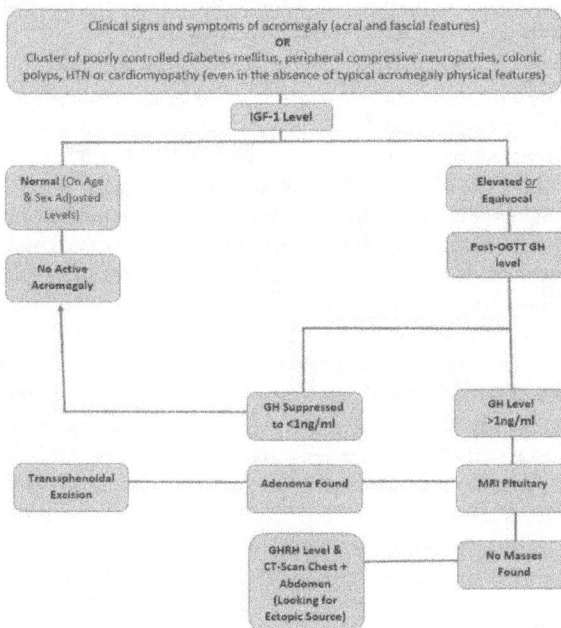

Figure 3.
Acromegaly diagnosis algorithm.

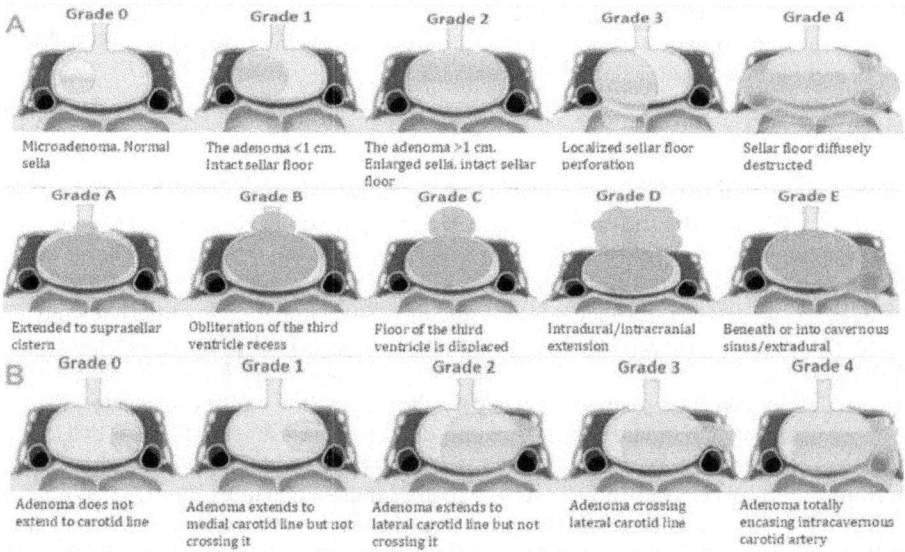

Figure 4.
Modified Hardy's classification for sphenoidal sinus and extrasellar extension (A), and Knosp classification of cavernous sinus invasion (B).

6.3 Management

The goal of management in GH-secreting adenomas is to normalize GH/IGF-1 levels, remove the mass effect of adenoma from surrounding neurovascular structure, and reverse or control comorbidities that are related to high GH levels. Most of biochemical and structural changes caused by high GH status are reversible (**Table 5**). Treated acromegaly patients with postoperative GH <1 ng/mL have mortality rate that is similar to age-matched general population [27].

Surgical excision through a trans-sphenoidal route is the gold standard. Unless it is contraindicated, all patients should be offered surgical excision of the adenoma. In older reports before the year of 2000, GH normalization rate after surgical management was between 40 and 70% [28]. The most common cause of incomplete tumor excision and failure of GH normalization after surgery is extra-sellar tumor growth, specifically invasion into the cavernous sinus. Adenoma total resection will result in a biochemical cure which is defined as IGF-1 within normal range for age and gender, and suppression of GH to <1 ng/mL following OGTT [29].

Recent studies have found that the rate of medial wall invasion in GH-secreting adenomas between 70 and 89% and resection of the medial wall of the cavernous sinus resulted in higher post-operative GH normalization rate which in recent reports was found to be 67–92% [29–32]. Detection of suprasellar extension or cavernous sinus invasion can be evaluated and graded on pre-operative MRI scans by using Hardy's and Knops' classification systems (**Figure 4**), This system uses CISS and VIPE sequences to evaluate cavernous sinus invasion and optic canal tumor extension [33, 34].

Treatment algorithm is summarized in (**Figure 5**) which is adopted from The Endocrine Society Guidelines released in 2014 [35].

Important points regarding the management of GH-secreting adenomas:

- Surgical debulking should be offered to patients who harbor large adenomas with significant extra-sellar extension as that would increase the response to medical therapy.

Cardiovascular changes	Outcome	Notes
Hypertrophic cardiomyopathy	Reversable	Better prognosis in patients <40 years and shorter duration of GH exposure (<5 years duration)
Arrhythmias	Reversable	
Hypertension	Possible reversable	Unsolid data showed possible reversibility
Valvular hear disease	Irreversible	Mitral and aortic valves are most commonly affected
Metabolic changes	**Outcome**	**Notes**
Insulin resistance/ diabetes	Reversable	Depends on the status of beta-cells function. *Octreotide* associated with deleterious effect on glucose metabolism especially at the beginning of treatment
Hyperlipidemia	Reversable	
Respiratory changes	**Outcome**	**Notes**
Sleep apnea	Reversible (unless significant remodeling of upper airways due to long-standing acromegaly)	Nocturnal PEEP-ventilation assisted device ma needed in treated patients with irreversible upper airway changes
Lung volume and elasticity	Reversible	
Musculoskeletal changes	**Outcome**	**Notes**
Arthropathy	Irreversible	Treated patients may have improvement on pain and range of motion, but not on the structural joints changes.
Carpal tunnel syndrome	Reversible	

Table 5.
Reversible and irreversible biochemical and structural changes in treated acromegaly patients [22].

- All patients who had total resection of the adenoma and achieved biochemical cure should be followed-up with IGF-1 level annually.

- All patients who did not achieve biochemical cure should be treated with octreotide (SRL). Pegvisomant is added to medical regimen if the response on octreotide is suboptimal.

- Radiotherapy is offered for patients who had recurrent adenoma or in sub-optimal response on medical therapy. All patient who received radiotherapy should be monitored for hypopituitarism as 80–100% of patients will develop it about 10 years after radiotherapy [28]. It is particularly helpful in adenoma growth control in 90% of patients and can achieve normal IGF-1 level in up to 70% of patients, however, full response takes 10 to 15 years to be seen [28, 36].

- On early morning of post-operative day 1, GH level < 2 ng/ml is highly predictive of surgical biochemical cure [37].

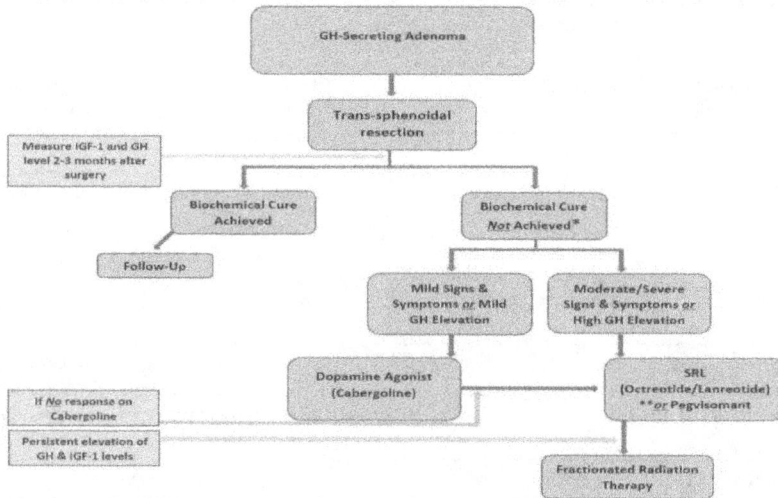

Figure 5.
Acromegaly management algorithm. SRL, somatostatin receptors ligands. *Repeat surgery is recommended for residual and resectable disease. **SRL are the first line of management in patients who are poor surgical candidates, have extensive parasellar invasion, or who had only tumor debulking.

- Octreotide may result in gastrointestinal hypomotility and increase the risk of gallbladder stones, however, regular monitoring with ultrasound is not needed.

- Pegvisomant reversibly elevates liver enzymes. Patients should have liver enzymes monitored every month for first 6 months and every 6 months thereafter. If liver enzymes become elevated three-times above the baseline level, Pegvisomant should be stopped.

- Patients may experience excessive diuresis after surgery with immediate improvement in soft tissue edema which should be differentiated from postoperative diabetes insipidus. This phenomenon occurs due to fluid mobilization from soft tissue as GH cause significant fluid retention and plasma volume expansion. Zada et al. found that patients with a negative cumulative fluid balance at 48 hours after surgery were more than twice as likely to have a GH level of <1.5 ng/ml (55 vs. 25%, p = 0.023) [38].

7. Cushing disease

Cushing disease (CD) is a clinical syndrome caused by exposure to supraphysiological levels of cortisol due to adrenocorticotropic hormone (ACTH) hypersecretion from pituitary gland. Cushing disease has an annual incidence of about 2.4 cases/million and a prevalence of 39.1 cases/million [39, 40]. The cause of 70% of endogenous CD is by pituitary adenomas. 20–30% of endogenous CD are due to ectopic-ACTH secreting tumors, 50% of them are from lung cancer.

In normal physiological conditions, ACTH secretion from the anterior pituitary gland is under stimulatory effect by corticotropin-releasing hormone (CRH) released from the paraventricular hypothalamic nucleus. CRH is delivered to pituitary corticotroph cells through hypophyseal portal venous system. ACTH release will stimulate cortisol secretion from adrenal glands. Cortisol will exert an inhibitory effect on ACTH and CRH release from pituitary gland and the hypothalamic nucleus, respectively, in a negative feedback-mechanism. Adenoma cells are not sensitive to high levels of cortisol, however, CRH levels will be suppressed.

ACTH-secreting adenomas are rare, they constitute around 6% of pituitary adenomas [41]. On diagnosis, the majority are microadenomas and only 4–10% are macroadenomas [40]. Unlike acromegaly, CD has female predominance (3:1). Unlike prolactinomas and GH-secreting adenomas, ACTH-secreting adenomas have no relationship between the size of the adenoma and the extent of hypersecretion. Mathioudakis et al. found that patients with microadenomas had more clinical signs and symptoms overall when compared to patients with macroadenomas [42].

7.1 Clinical presentation

High cortisol levels have deleterious effects on almost every organ or system in the body. The most common signs and symptoms are glucose intolerance, hypertension, plethoric rounded facies, decreased libido in both sexes, and menstrual irregularities in females [43]. Other manifestations include osteoporosis, skin thinning and easy bruising, buffalo hump, acne, and proximal muscle weakness. In the pediatric age group, CD should be suspected in children who present with rapid weight gain, growth retardation and dorsocervical fat pad. Uncontrolled CD is associated with high mortality with estimated 5 years' survival of 50% [44]. The main causes of morbidity and mortality in untreated patient are myocardial infarction, strokes, diabetes mellitus, and infection. However, even after successful management, patients are at higher risk for lethal cardiovascular incidents up to 5 years after treatment [45].

7.2 Evaluation

Early recognition of CD is vital for mitigation of long-term consequences from high cortisol exposure. The first step in diagnosis relies on clinical suspicion. Exogenous corticosteroid source should be first ruled-out by a detailed history. The diagnostic work-up is summarized by 3 broad steps: detection of high cortisol level, ACTH level status, and localization of the disease origin (**Figure 6**). After biochemical confirmation of Cushing syndrome, ACTH level should be measured.

Low-ACTH levels mean that pituitary cells are suppressed and there is no extra-pituitary ACTH secretion. In this setting, it is prudent to rule-out adrenal adenomas. If ACTH level is high, CD is confirmed and the localization of the source of ACTH secretion should be evaluated. Unlike cancer cells that secret ACTH, adenomas affecting corticotrophic pituitary cells are usually suppressed by exogenous high corticosteroids doses. High-dose dexamethasone test (e.g. 8 mg given at 9 p.m. and cortisol levels measured at 8 a.m. the next morning) will suppress ACTH secreted from pituitary adenoma but not from ectopic sources. MRI pituitary need to be ordered if high-dose dexamethasone test localize the source to pituitary gland. As mentioned earlier, 70–75% of ACTH-secreting adenomas are microadenomas. However, up to 60% of these adenomas are not detected on MRI [43, 45, 46]. To increase detection rate of the adenoma, volumetric interpolated breath-hold examination (VIBE) sequences should be added [47]. If the brain MRI is negative or high-dose dexamethasone test is unequivocal and a pituitary source is still highly suspected, inferior petrosal sinus (IPS) sampling would confirm the pituitary source and also localize the tumor within the pituitary gland to the left or right side. IPS sampling has an accuracy rate of up to 95%, however, it is an invasive procedure and requires highly experienced operators. To enhance the detection rate, bilateral simultaneous IPS sampling after CRH *or* desmopressin stimulation is highly recommended (**Figure 7**) [48, 49].

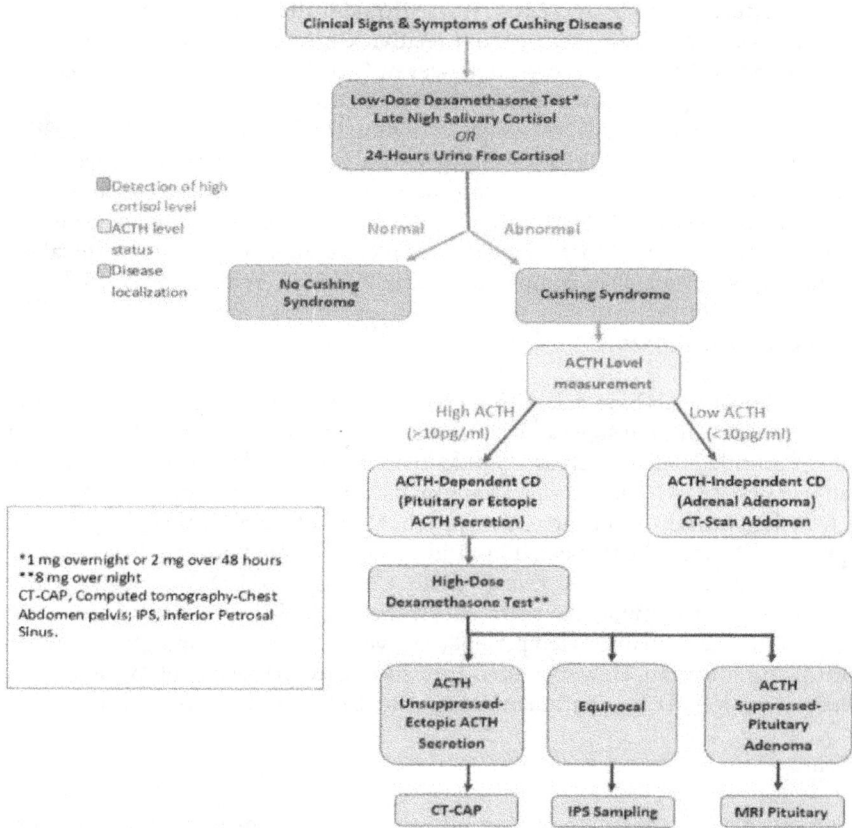

Figure 6.
Diagnosis algorithm for Cushing disease.

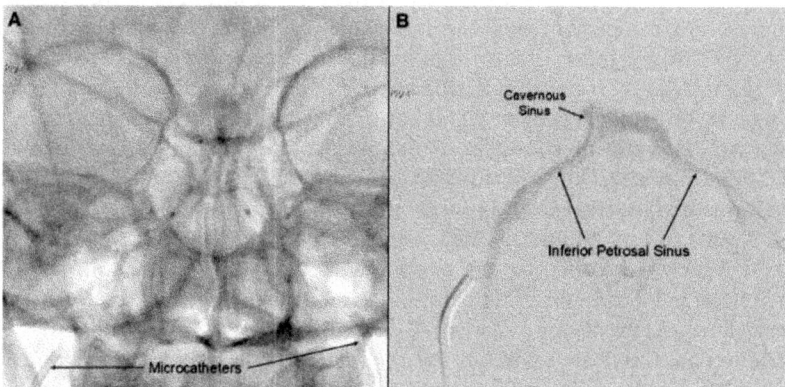

Figure 7.
Bilateral internal jugular vein catheterization (A) and selective contrast injection and sampling of bilateral inferior petrosal sinuses (B).

It is important to mention that IPS sampling is not recommended for adenoma localization in previous surgically treated patients because the venous drainage of the pituitary gland lateralizes unpredictably after initial surgery [50].

7.3 Management

The only current treatment is surgery, and the aim should be total adenomectomy. Surgical cure and recurrence rate depends on surgeon experience, adenoma size, extra-sellar extension, and adenoma detection on preoperative MRI. The definition of postoperative biochemical remission varies in the literature but cortisol levels in the early morning after surgery <5 µg/dl within 2–7 days of adenomectomy is widely considered to have high positive predictive value of remission [51].

Remission rate in surgically treated CD is 69–93% [52–54]. Recurrence rate after successful management is between 3 and 22% of patients after 3 years [50]. However, in patients whose preoperative MRI failed to show the adenoma, remission rate drops to 50–70% [54]. Adenomectomy resection using pseudocapsule technique in which the tumor is resected with its surrounding adherent pituitary cells is associated with higher success rate, longer remission rate, and higher rate of cortisol decline in the post-operative period (**Figure 8**) [45, 55].

In cases where the adenoma is small or not visualized on MRI, several options are available which will aid in intraoperative tumor localization. Waston et al. could localize ACTH-secreting adenomas by using intraoperative ultrasound in 69% of their patients with negative preoperative MRI [56]. If intraoperative ultrasound is not available or inconclusive, sellar exploration with making multiple cuts within the pituitary gland looking for the adenoma may be warranted. However, in such cases it is very important to expose the whole pituitary gland by wide removal of sellar floor bone and wide dural opening. Additionally, it is crucial to expose the anterior and medial walls of cavernous sinuses bilaterally for adequate visualization. If the exploration was not fruitful, then a partial hypophysectomy of the side that was lateralized by IPS sampling should be considered. Total hypophysectomy (i.e. removal of the anterior pituitary gland while leaving the posterior gland attached to the stalk) may be considered in cases where IPS sampling was unable to lateralize the adenoma, or in cases where intraoperative localization of the adenoma failed.

But the question is when to consider that patient has failed the surgical management and did not achieve remission?

Determining when to consider a patient has failed surgical management is difficult. As stated, all patients should have their cortisol levels evaluated the morning

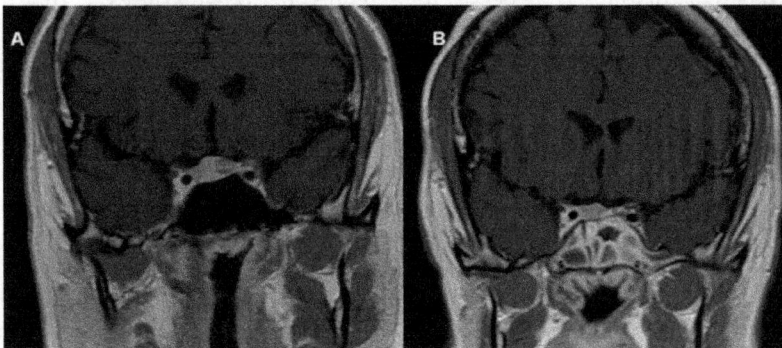

Figure 8.
A 30-year-old female patient presented with typical features of Cushing disease. Preoperative workup revealed high cortisol level. She was investigated with MRI pituitary with contrast which showed microadenoma involving the left half of the pituitary gland (A). The patient underwent endoscopic transsphenoidal total resection by utilizing pseudocapsular technique (B). She went to complete remission 36 hours after surgery.

after surgery. Immediate postoperative cortisol levels may fluctuate. Generally after 72 h, cortisol level is stabilized, and therefore can be a better determinant of whether that the patient did not reach the remission state [57]. However, it was found that cortisol level ≤2 µg/dl within first 24 h after surgery there is a 100% sensitivity for durable remission [58]. A serum cortisol value >5 µg/dl up to 6 weeks post-surgery is considered to have persistent disease and should be considered for repeat surgery. Ten percent of patients who had durable remission after adenomectomy will develop recurrence of the disease, therefore, all patients need regular long follow-up for recurrence monitoring [59].

Then, what if the patient failed first surgery and remission did not achieved?

If a patient failed to achieve remission after their first surgery, it is always advisable to do an exploration of the pituitary gland and resect any remnant of the adenoma. Firstly, a pituitary MRI should be repeated; if MRI shows remnant adenoma, resection is needed as soon as possible. If MRI failed to show the remnant disease, surgical exploration of the resected cavity and possible partial or total hypophysectomy should be considered.

But, what if partial or total hypophysectomy have been done in first operation?

In such cases, patient should receive medical therapy, radiotherapy, or other adjuvant therapy.

The aforementioned plan can also be adopted for recurrent disease after an initial biochemical cure. In terms of radiotherapy, stereotactic radiosurgery has the highest incidence of CD remission with rate of 70–75% according to recent reports [60, 61].

Most patients who had successful resection of the adenoma will develop hypocortisolism. This is happens due to longstanding suppression of normal corticotroph cells by high cortisol levels and it takes more than 6 months for those cells to recover. In our practice, we do the first cortisol level measurement 6 h after the surgery and we repeat it every 6 h for the first 3 days. We give replacement therapy (hydrocortisone 8 mg/m^2 on early morning and 4 mg/m^2 on evening) only if cortisol level < 1.8 ug/dl. Hypopituitarism occurs after adenoma resection in <5% of cases, therefore, pituitary function assessment should be usually done 2 weeks after surgery by measuring prolactin and T4 levels [45].

Lastly, Cushing's disease patients have an increased risk of venous thromboembolism (VTE). The incidence of postoperative VTE was found to be 3.4% in one study. Excess circulating corticosteroids cause inhibition of fibrinolysis and accelerated activation of coagulation factors. Even after correction of high cortisol level, Hypercoagulability state persist for extended period and the exact time of hemostatic parameters normalization is not well studied [62]. One proposed plan is to keep the VTE chemoprophylaxis up to 30 days after surgery [62].

8. Nonfunctional pituitary adenoma

Non-functional, or non-secretory, adenomas constitute about 10–20% of all intracranial tumors and 15–30% of all pituitary adenomas [63]. They are the second most common pituitary adenoma after prolactinoma. However, if only macroadenomas are considered, NFPA is the most common one [64]. NFPA is unique compared to functional pituitary adenomas in different aspects. First, NFPA are usually seen in old age groups compared to functional adenomas. Second, patients present mainly with signs and symptoms of mass effect. Third, large number of patients have hypopituitarism in one or more of pituitary axes. On the other side, many of NFPA patients are detected incidentally (pituitary incidentalomas). The incidence of asymptomatic NFPA varies in the literature, but one large meta-analysis-autopsy study found the mean prevalence of pituitary incidentalomas was 10.7% [65].

The natural history of incidentally discovered NFPA remains relatively unknown. However, the risk of tumor expansion is related closely to tumor size on presentation and, to lesser extent, tumor relation to optic apparatus [66]. Microadenomas have a low chance of expansion (19%) compared to macroadenomas (25–50% of macroadenoma patients show tumor expansion on follow-up imaging) [66].

8.1 Clinical presentation

The most common presentation of NFPA is headache. It may be caused by intrasellar pressure increment and dural lining compression which are innervated by trigeminal nerve branches. Visual field defect is the second most common clinical presentation that may be seen in up to 61% of cases [64, 67]. Visual field defects are asymmetrical in 2/3 of the patients. They occur due to optic nerves and/or chiasm displacement and compression, which also may result in permanent deficit in long-standing compressions.

Tumor extension to cavernous sinus may result in ophthalmoplegia due to compression of CNIII, CNIV, and CNVI. CNIII is most commonly affected followed by CNVI and then CNIV.

Adenomas greater than >4 cm of diameter may obstruct foramen of Monro and cause obstructive hydrocephalus.

Pituitary apoplexy is another common presentation for these lesions. Pituitary apoplexy is most commonly seen in NFPA, accounting for 45–82% of pituitary apoplexy cases, and 7–9.5% of asymptomatic NFPA present initially with pituitary apoplexy [64].

Hypopituitarism is another common sequela of NFPA. 70–85% patients will have deficiency in at least one axis of pituitary cells secretion [68]. Hypopituitarism occurs in an expected sequence of hormonal loss which usually affect GH, then LF/FSH, then TSH, and lastly ACTH. Diabetes insipidus is rare in non-surgically-NFPA-treated patients, and if it is found in a patient with pituitary lesion, other lesions should be considered (e.g. craniopharyngioma, aneurysms, metastasis).

Lastly, as stated previously, NFPA may be discovered incidentally on brain MRI that was done for other causes. In one large single-center prospective study, 49% of NFPA presented incidentally and 85% of them harbored macroadenomas. Interestingly, in the same cohort, they found that half of the patients in the asymptomatic group reported some mass effects symptoms like headache and/or visual symptoms and only 35% of the incidentally discovered group (in which brain imaging done for unrelated reasons) has no symptoms at all [69].

8.2 Evaluation

All patients who their imaging studies showed pituitary adenoma, whether symptomatic or asymptomatic, should go thorough hormonal evaluation as recommended by The Clinical Guidelines Subcommittee of The Endocrine Society [70]. These include IGF-1 and GH, ACTH, prolactin, FSH/LH, and TSH. If ACTH and IGF-1 test are equivocal, stimulatory tests are recommended. Hypopituitarism is not uncommon and hormonal replacement therapy should be initiated in patients with hormonal deficiency. Panhypopituitarism can be seen in up to 30% of patients. Prolactin level could be elevated in 25–65% caused by pituitary stalk compression (stalk effect) [71]. Therefore, it is important to differentiate between hyperprolactinemia caused by a prolactinoma or NFPA. Prolactin level > 200 µg/L is unlikely to be caused by stalk effect.

The diagnostic approach and follow-up are different between symptomatic and asymptomatic NFPA. In symptomatic NFPA, and after doing the hormonal laboratory tests, all patients need to have ophthalmic evaluation for assessing optic apparatus

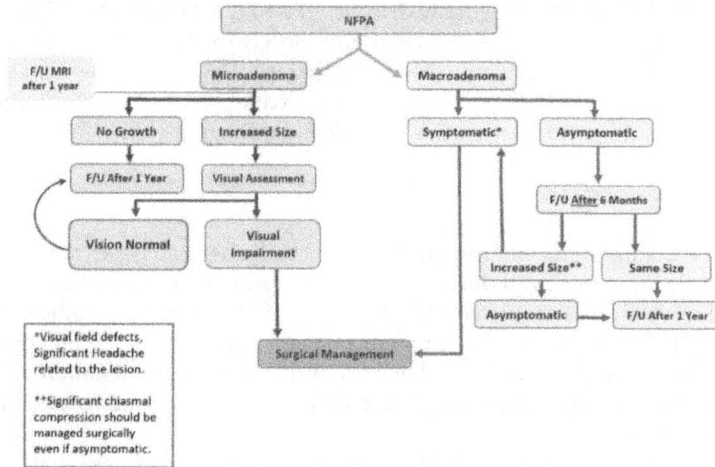

Figure 9.
Simplified scheme of NFPA diagnosis and management.

function. Also, it is important to have a detailed history and physical examination to assess the patient symptoms. In asymptomatic NFPA, patients need to have complete hormonal evaluation as mentioned previously to rule-out hyper-or-hypopituitarism. Asymptomatic microadenomas can be followed-up after 1 year of diagnosis by repeating the brain imaging only. In asymptomatic macroadenomas, follow-up is after 6 months with brain MRI and hormone levels, then every year if the follow-up images and laboratories did not show tumor progression or pituitary dysfunction (**Figure 9**).

8.3 Management

Treatment of patients with NFPA starts with hormonal replacement therapy in case of hypopituitarism. It is vital to recognize and treat cortisol deficiency efficiently. The same is true for secondary hypothyroidism as patients should receive thyroxine immediately after confirming its deficiency. Both cortisol and thyroxine should be initiated before surgery, and in non-emergency surgery, it is better to replace thyroxine and wait until hypothyroidism is adequately treated.

Surgical indications for NFPA are symptomatic optic nerve or chiasm compression, cranial nerves dysfunction, and pituitary apoplexy with visual impairment (**Figure 9**). However, surgery is also advised in asymptomatic growing adenomas that are close to or progressively abutting optic nerves and/or chiasm on follow-up imaging studies [70].

What about patients who have hypopituitarism or headache only?

Surgery in patients with hypopituitarism alone without visual symptoms is not recommended as only 30% of patients will have improvement over pituitary function. Also, headache is a common symptom in NFPA patients, but as headache has multiple causes, there is a high chance of headache persistence after adenoma resection. Therefore, only intractable headache that is affecting patient's daily activities should be an indication of surgery and the patient should be aware that headache relief cannot be guaranteed [71].

After surgery, patients should be evaluated for hypopituitarism 6 weeks after surgery. Also, pituitary MRI should be done 3 months after surgery to have it as a baseline for future follow-up. Gross-total resection of NFPA has a recurrence rate of 7–24%, and 47–64% of cases in partially resected ones [72].

9. Surgical approaches to pituitary adenomas

Currently, pituitary adenomas are approached almost exclusively through transsphenoidal route because it offers a direct access to sellar and suprasellar region by removing of posterior wall of sphenoidal sinus. Also, it is associated with lower morbidity and it is considered a less invasive approach than the transcranial route. Either endoscopic and microscopic, transsphenoidal approach is adequate to remove intrasellar lesions with satisfactory outcomes. Recent advancements in surgical endoscopy have improved our ability to visualize and dissect normal anatomical structures from the adherent pathologies in a way that is nearly similar to microneurosurgery. However, in selected cases, transcranial approaches are still needed for resecting tumors extending to suprasellar or parasellar regions that could not be addressed by transsphenoidal approaches.

9.1 Transsphenoidal approach

It is an extra-arachnoidal direct route to pituitary gland. It has the advantage of avoiding brain retraction, early optic nerves decompression with minimal manipulation, and wide operative view. Posterior wall of sphenoidal sinus, or sellar floor, can be accessed via a transnasal or translabial route. Usually, it involves the usage of microscope, endoscope, or both. Whether endoscope or microscope is used, the procedure has three-stages that are needed to reach the intrasellar space: nasal stage, sphenoidal stage, and sellar stage.

It is important to utilize an operative setup that is comfortable for whole team. Patient is typically positioned supine with 20-degrees head elevation and is positioned straight or slightly extended and fixed using Mayfield head clamp. The surgeon usually operates on the right and facing of the patient. We prefer to have the scrub nurse on the right side of the surgeon and the assistant on the left side. The screen and the navigation are positioned on the left side of the patient facing the surgeon (**Figure 10**). Neuronavigation is essential for dealing with tumors that extended to supra- or para-sellar regions, and recurrent tumors.

9.1.1 Nasal stage

Using 0-degree endoscopy, inferior, middle and superior turbinates are identified. Middle turbinate usually obstructs the access to sphenoidal sinus. To have unobstructed route, middle turbinate is typically displaced laterally, or resected if a wider view is needed, using a blunt dissector to create enough working space. After that, the choana is found on the inferomedial aspect of the view. Sphenoethmoidal

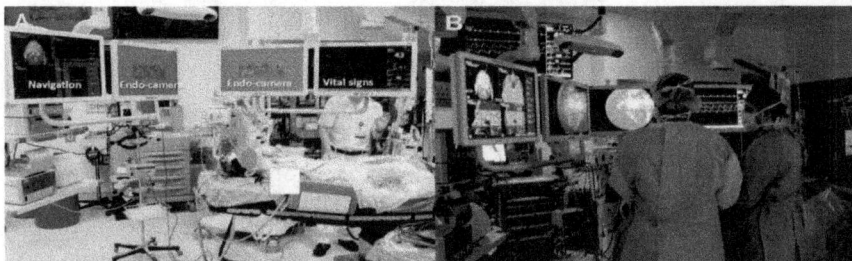

Figure 10.
Patient positioned supine, with head slightly extended, monitors are placed to left of the patient (A).
The surgeon standing on the right of the patient and the assistant on the surgeon's left side (B).

recess is identified and sphenoid ostium is seen on the roof of the recess and the choana. Nasal septum the best landmark for midline identification.

9.1.2 Sphenoidal stage

It starts with enlarging the sphenoidal ostium lateral and inferiorly. This step is usually undertaken by using chisel or high-speed drill. Care is taken to avoid injury to sphenopalatine artery the lies in the inferolateral direction. Posterior nasal septum is coagulated and detached from the sphenoidal rostrum. Anterior wall of the sphenoidal sinus now is exposed, circumferentially with bony removal using high-speed drill and sphenoidal rostrum is removed in fragments. It is important to perform a wide removal of anterior wall of sphenoidal sinus to avoid a narrow working space. Multiple sphenoidal septa can be seen inside the sinus and may need to be drilled. Care is taken septa drilling as one or more of the septa may be attached to carotid prominences.

9.1.3 Sellar stage

After a wide removal of anterior wall of sphenoidal sinus and drilling of sphenoidal septa, sellar floor will be seen. Important anatomical landmarks at sellar floor include carotids, optic nerves, pituitary prominences, and lateral opticocarotid recesses bilaterally (**Figure 2**). Progressive thinning of sellar floor using diamond drill and Kerrison rongeur till the dura over the pituitary gland is exposed. Lateral and superior exposure depends on the extent of the tumor. We prefer not to expose the intracavernous carotids unless the anterior wall of cavernous sinus is needed to be opened for medial wall resection or when dealing with functional adenomas.

9.1.4 Complications

Transsphenoidal approach is usually safe and associated with low morbidity rate [73]. The most feared intraoperative complication is ICA injury, which has a very low incidence rate. However, it is associated with significant morbidity and mortality. Consequences of a such injury include pseudoaneurysm formation and carotid cavernous fistula.

Postoperative complications include the ones related to the nose (nasal septum perforation, insomnia, epistaxis from injury to sphenopalatine artery or its branches), sphenoid sinus complications (mucocele formation, sinusitis or sphenoid bone fractures), or related to intrasellar (hemorrhage, cerebrospinal fluid (CSF) leak and tension pneumocephalus).

CSF leak incidence has decreased in recent years due to the advancements and newer techniques in harvesting vascularized nasoseptal flaps [74]. CSF leak incidence in recently published series falls between 1% and 4% [75].

9.2 Transcranial approaches

The majority of patients can be treated using transsphenoidal route. However, a few of pituitary adenomas may require transcranial approaches for resecting adenoma extensions that cannot be reached by transsphenoidal route.

Common indications for transcranial surgery in pituitary adenomas include:

1. Lateral and significant suprasellar adenoma extensions to critical neurovascular structures.

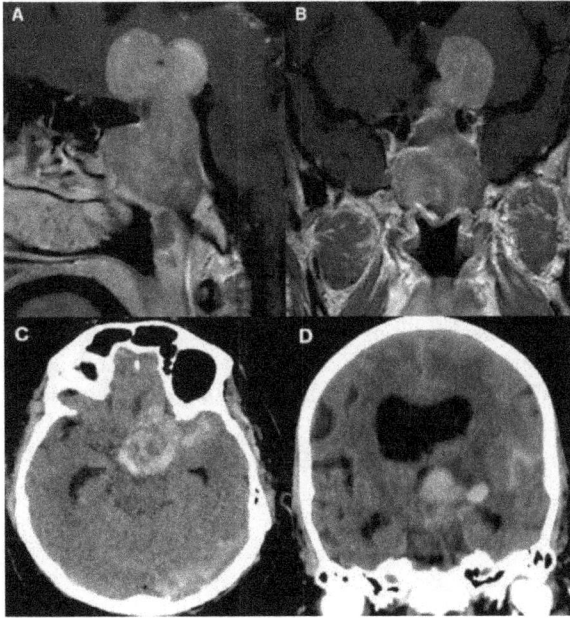

Figure 11.
Preoperative MRI (A and B) and postoperative CT scan (C and D) for a senior male patient who was complaining form headache and progressive visual dysfunction. The patient was operated in outside hospital through transsphenoidal approach. Incomplete excision was done. However, the patient developed decrease in the level of consciousness and oculomotor nerve dysfunction after surgery. Brain CT scan showed excessive hemorrhage in the unresected intracranial part of the adenoma.

2. Anatomical challenges like conchal-type sphenoidal sinus, kissing carotids, sinuses infection.

3. Unsuccessful previous transsphenoidal surgery.

Other uncommon indications include patients with obstructive sleep apnea who could not be weaned off CPAP or concomitant aneurysm that is in proximity to the sellar area.

Recurrent adenomas are no longer an indication for transcranial surgery [76, 77]. Also, giant adenomas (>4 cm) used to be an indication for transcranial surgery, but due to recent advancements in endoscopic approaches, large size adenomas can be effectively treated through transsphenoidal route [78].

In dealing with giant pituitary adenomas that encasing nearby neurovascular structures, both transsphenoidal and transcranial may be needed, especially when the goal of surgery is gross total excision in functional-adenoma cases.

But what approach should be the first choice, the transsphenoidal or the transcranial surgery?

The answer of this question relies on the understanding of the blood supply of pituitary adenomas. These tumors share the same blood supply of normal pituitary gland which comes from inferior and superior hypophyseal arteries. In general, pituitary adenomas have low vascular density which may explain their slow growth [77]. Attacking the adenoma through transsphenoidal route will result in acute devascularization of the remaining unresected adenoma which result in intratumoral necrosis and subsequently hemorrhage (**Figure 11**). Therefore, it is preferred to go transcranially first then to operate transsphenoidal [79, 80].

Transcranial approaches that commonly utilized to deal with pituitary adenomas include pterional, orbitozygomatic, bifrontal, and supraorbital approaches. The choice of the approach depends on tumor extension and the neurovascular structures that are needed to be addressed intraoperatively.

10. Conclusion

Pituitary adenomas associated with significant morbidity and require multiple modalities of treatment. Management is usually surgical except for prolactinomas. The therapeutic decision should be adjusted to adenomas type, center expertise, and patient desire. Thorough understanding of the pathophysiology and management options of PA different types is essential to achieve the therapeutic goals, which can be summarized in pituitary and neurological function restoration.

Author details

Bilal Ibrahim, Mauricio Mandel, Assad Ali, Edinson Najera, Michal Obrzut, Badih Adada and Hamid Borghei-Razavi*
Department of Neurosurgery, Braathen Center, Cleveland Clinic Florida, Weston, Florida, USA

*Address all correspondence to: borgheh2@ccf.org

IntechOpen

References

[1] Ostrom QT, Cioffi G, Waite K, Kruchko C, Barnholtz-Sloan JS. CBTRUS statistical report: Primary brain and other central nervous system tumors diagnosed in the United States in 2014-2018. Neuro-Oncology. 2021;**23**(12 Suppl 2):iii1-iii105. DOI: 10.1093/neuonc/noab200

[2] Perry A, Graffeo CS, Marcellino C, Pollock BE, Wetjen NM, Meyer FB. Pediatric pituitary adenoma: Case series, review of the literature, and a Skull Base treatment paradigm. Journal of Neurological Surgery Part B. Skull Base. 2018;**79**(1):91-114. DOI: 10.1055/s-0038-1625984

[3] Aflorei ED, Korbonits M. Epidemiology and etiopathogenesis of pituitary adenomas. Journal of Neuro-Oncology. 2014;**117**(3):379-394. DOI: 10.1007/s11060-013-1354-5

[4] Truong HQ, Borghei-Razavi H, Najera E, et al. Bilateral coagulation of inferior hypophyseal artery and pituitary transposition during endoscopic endonasal interdural posterior clinoidectomy: Do they affect pituitary function? Journal of Neurosurgery. 2018;**131**(1):141-146. DOI: 10.3171/2018.2.JNS173126

[5] Hall WA, Luciano MG, Doppman JL, Patronas NJ, Oldfield EH. Pituitary magnetic resonance imaging in normal human volunteers: Occult adenomas in the general population. Annals of Internal Medicine. 1994;**120**(10):817-820. DOI: 10.7326/0003-4819-120-10-199405150-00001

[6] Jho DH, Biller BM, Agarwalla PK, Swearingen B. Pituitary apoplexy: Large surgical series with grading system. World Neurosurgery. 2014;**82**(5):781-790. DOI: 10.1016/j.wneu.2014.06.005

[7] Johnston PC, Hamrahian AH, Weil RJ, Kennedy L. Pituitary tumor apoplexy. Journal of Clinical Neuroscience. 2015;**22**(6):939-944. DOI: 10.1016/j.jocn.2014.11.023. Epub 2015 Mar 20

[8] Baker HL Jr. The angiographic delineation of sellar and parasellar masses. Radiology. 1972;**104**(1):67-78. DOI: 10.1148/104.1.67

[9] Randeva HS, Schoebel J, Byrne J, Esiri M, Adams CB, Wass JA. Classical pituitary apoplexy: Clinical features, management and outcome. Clinical Endocrinology. 1999;**51**(2):181-188. DOI: 10.1046/j.1365-2265.1999.00754.x

[10] Kasantikul V, Shuangshoti S. Pituitary adenomas: Immunohistochemical: Study of 90 cases. Journal of the Medical Association of Thailand. 1990;**73**(9):514-521

[11] Casanueva FF, Molitch ME, Schlechte JA, et al. Guidelines of the pituitary society for the diagnosis and management of prolactinomas. Clinical Endocrinology. 2006;**65**(2):265-273. DOI: 10.1111/j.1365-2265.2006.02562.x

[12] Schlechte JA. Clinical practice. Prolactinoma. New England Journal of Medicine. 2003;**349**(21):2035-2041. DOI: 10.1056/NEJMcp025334

[13] Schlechte J, Dolan K, Sherman B, Chapler F, Luciano A. The natural history of untreated hyperprolactinemia: A prospective analysis. The Journal of Clinical Endocrinology and Metabolism. 1989;**68**(2):412-418. DOI: 10.1210/jcem-68-2-412

[14] Bevan JS, Webster J, Burke CW, Scanlon MF. Dopamine agonists and pituitary tumor shrinkage. Endocrine Reviews. 1992;**13**(2):220-240. DOI: 10.1210/edrv-13-2-220

[15] Molitch ME. Pregnancy and the hyperprolactinemic woman. The New

England Journal of Medicine. 1985;**312**(21):1364-1370. DOI: 10.1056/NEJM198505233122106

[16] Konopka P, Raymond JP, Merceron RE, Seneze J. Continuous administration of bromocriptine in the prevention of neurological complications in pregnant women with prolactinomas. American Journal of Obstetrics and Gynecology. 1983;**146**(8):935-938. DOI: 10.1016/0002-9378(83)90968-7

[17] Smith TR, Hulou MM, Huang KT, et al. Current indications for the surgical treatment of prolactinomas. Journal of Clinical Neuroscience. 2015;**22**(11):1785-1791. DOI: 10.1016/j.jocn.2015.06.001

[18] Liuzzi A, Dallabonzana D, Oppizzi G, et al. Low doses of dopamine agonists in the long-term treatment of macroprolactinomas. The New England Journal of Medicine. 1985;**313**(11):656-659. DOI: 10.1056/NEJM198509123131103

[19] Holdaway IM, Rajasoorya C. Epidemiology of acromegaly. Pituitary. 1999;**2**(1):29-41. DOI: 10.1023/a:1009965803750

[20] Mazziotti G, Bianchi A, Bonadonna S, et al. Prevalence of vertebral fractures in men with acromegaly. The Journal of Clinical Endocrinology and Metabolism. 2008;**93**(12):4649-4655. DOI: 10.1210/jc.2008-0791

[21] Colao A, Ferone D, Marzullo P, Lombardi G. Systemic complications of acromegaly: Epidemiology, pathogenesis, and management. Endocrine Reviews. 2004;**25**(1):102-152. DOI: 10.1210/er.2002-0022

[22] Clayton RN. Cardiovascular function in acromegaly. Endocrine Reviews. 2003;**24**(3):272-277. DOI: 10.1210/er.2003-0009

[23] Maison P, Démolis P, Young J, Schaison G, Giudicelli JF, Chanson P. Vascular reactivity in acromegalic patients: Preliminary evidence for regional endothelial dysfunction and increased sympathetic vasoconstriction. Clinical Endocrinology. 2000;**53**(4):445-451. DOI: 10.1046/j.1365-2265.2000.01127.x

[24] Sughrue ME, Chang EF, Gabriel RA, Aghi MK, Blevins LS. Excess mortality for patients with residual disease following resection of pituitary adenomas. Pituitary. 2011;**14**(3):276-283. DOI: 10.1007/s11102-011-0308-1

[25] Delhougne B, Deneux C, Abs R, Chanson P, Fierens H, Laurent-Puig P, et al. The prevalence of colonic polyps in acromegaly: A colonoscopic and pathological study in 103 patients. The Journal of Clinical Endocrinology and Metabolism. 1995;**80**(11):3223-3226. DOI: 10.1210/jcem.80.11.7593429

[26] Cairns SR, Scholefield JH, Steele RJ, et al. Guidelines for colorectal cancer screening and surveillance in moderate and high risk groups (update from 2002). Gut. 2010;**59**(5):666-689. DOI: 10.1136/gut.2009.179804

[27] Holdaway IM, Rajasoorya RC, Gamble GD. Factors influencing mortality in acromegaly. The Journal of Clinical Endocrinology and Metabolism. 2004;**89**(2):667-674. DOI: 10.1210/jc.2003-031199

[28] Chanson P, Salenave S, Kamenicky P, Cazabat L, Young J. Pituitary tumours: Acromegaly. Best Practice & Research. Clinical Endocrinology & Metabolism. 2009;**23**(5):555-574. DOI: 10.1016/j.beem.2009.05.010

[29] Babu H, Ortega A, Nuno M, et al. Long-term endocrine outcomes following endoscopic endonasal transsphenoidal surgery for acromegaly and associated prognostic factors.

Neurosurgery. 2017;**81**(2):357-366. DOI: 10.1093/neuros/nyx020

[30] Nagata Y, Takeuchi K, Yamamoto T, et al. Removal of the medial wall of the cavernous sinus for functional pituitary adenomas: A technical report and pathologic significance. World Neurosurgery. 2019;**126**:53-58. DOI: 10.1016/j.wneu.2019.02.134

[31] Cohen-Cohen S, Gardner PA, Alves-Belo JT, et al. The medial wall of the cavernous sinus. Part 2: Selective medial wall resection in 50 pituitary adenoma patients. Journal of Neurosurgery. 2018;**131**(1):131-140. DOI: 10.3171/2018.5.JNS18595

[32] Nishioka H, Fukuhara N, Horiguchi K, Yamada S. Aggressive transsphenoidal resection of tumors invading the cavernous sinus in patients with acromegaly: Predictive factors, strategies, and outcomes. Journal of Neurosurgery. 2014;**121**(3):505-510. DOI: 10.3171/2014.3.JNS132214

[33] Lang M, Silva D, Dai L, Kshettry VR, Woodard TD, Sindwani R, Recinos PF. Superiority of constructive interference in steady-state MRI sequencing over T1-weighted MRI sequencing for evaluating cavernous sinus invasion by pituitary macroadenomas. Journal of Neurosurgery JNS. 2019;**130**(2):352-359. DOI: 10.3171/2017.9.JNS171699

[34] Borghei-Razavi H, Lee J, Ibrahim B, et al. Accuracy and interrater reliability of CISS versus contrast-enhanced T1-weighted VIBE for the presence of optic canal invasion in tuberculum sellae meningiomas. World Neurosurgery. 2021;**148**:e502-e507. DOI: 10.1016/j.wneu.2021.01.015

[35] Katznelson L, Laws ER Jr, Melmed S, et al. Acromegaly: An endocrine society clinical practice guideline. The Journal of Clinical Endocrinology and Metabolism. 2014;**99**(11):3933-3951. DOI: 10.1210/jc.2014-2700

[36] Giustina A, Barkhoudarian G, Beckers A, et al. Multidisciplinary management of acromegaly: A consensus. Reviews in Endocrine & Metabolic Disorders. 2020;**21**(4):667-678. DOI: 10.1007/s11154-020-09588-z

[37] Krieger MD, Couldwell WT, Weiss MH. Assessment of long-term remission of acromegaly following surgery. Journal of Neurosurgery. 2003;**98**(4):719-724. DOI: 10.3171/jns.2003.98.4.0719

[38] Zada G, Sivakumar W, Fishback D, Singer PA, Weiss MH. Significance of postoperative fluid diuresis in patients undergoing transsphenoidal surgery for growth hormone-secreting pituitary adenomas. Journal of Neurosurgery. 2010;**112**(4):744-749. DOI: 10.3171/2009.7.JNS09438

[39] Etxabe J, Vazquez JA. Morbidity and mortality in Cushing's disease: An epidemiological approach. Clinical Endocrinology. 1994;**40**(4):479-484. DOI: 10.1111/j.1365-2265.1994.tb02486.x

[40] Woo YS, Isidori AM, Wat WZ, et al. Clinical and biochemical characteristics of adrenocorticotropin-secreting macroadenomas. The Journal of Clinical Endocrinology and Metabolism. 2005;**90**(8):4963-4969. DOI: 10.1210/jc.2005-0070

[41] Ntali G, Capatina C, Grossman A, Karavitaki N. Clinical review: Functioning gonadotroph adenomas. The Journal of Clinical Endocrinology and Metabolism. 2014;**99**(12):4423-4433. DOI: 10.1210/jc.2014-2362

[42] Mathioudakis N, Pendleton C, Quinones-Hinojosa A, Wand GS, Salvatori R. ACTH-secreting pituitary adenomas: Size does not correlate with hormonal activity. Pituitary. 2012;**15**(4):526-532. DOI: 10.1007/s11102-011-0362-8

[43] Newell-Price J, Trainer P, Besser M, Grossman A. The diagnosis and

differential diagnosis of Cushing's syndrome and pseudo-Cushing's states. Endocrine Reviews. 1998;**19**(5):647-672. DOI: 10.1210/edrv.19.5.0346

[44] Clayton RN, Raskauskiene D, Reulen RC, Jones PW. Mortality and morbidity in Cushing's disease over 50 years in Stoke-on-Trent, UK: Audit and meta-analysis of literature. The Journal of Clinical Endocrinology and Metabolism. 2011;**96**(3):632-642. DOI: 10.1210/jc.2010-1942

[45] Lonser RR, Nieman L, Oldfield EH. Cushing's disease: Pathobiology, diagnosis, and management. Journal of Neurosurgery. 2017;**126**(2):404-417. DOI: 10.3171/2016.1.JNS152119

[46] Invitti C, Pecori Giraldi F, de Martin M, Cavagnini F. Diagnosis and management of Cushing's syndrome: Results of an Italian multicentre study. Study Group of the Italian Society of Endocrinology on the Pathophysiology of the Hypothalamic-Pituitary-Adrenal Axis. The Journal of Clinical Endocrinology and Metabolism. 1999;**84**(2):440-448. DOI: 10.1210/jcem.84.2.5465

[47] Grober Y, Grober H, Wintermark M, Jane JA, Oldfield EH. Comparison of MRI techniques for detecting microadenomas in Cushing's disease. Journal of Neurosurgery. 2018;**128**(4):1051-1057. DOI: 10.3171/2017.3.JNS163122

[48] Kaltsas GA, Giannulis MG, Newell-Price JD, et al. A critical analysis of the value of simultaneous inferior petrosal sinus sampling in Cushing's disease and the occult ectopic adrenocorticotropin syndrome. The Journal of Clinical Endocrinology and Metabolism. 1999;**84**(2):487-492. DOI: 10.1210/jcem.84.2.5437

[49] Patil CG, Prevedello DM, Lad SP, et al. Late recurrences of Cushing's disease after initial successful transsphenoidal surgery. The Journal of Clinical Endocrinology and Metabolism. 2008;**93**(2):358-362. DOI: 10.1210/jc.2007-2013

[50] Rutkowski MJ, Flanigan PM, Aghi MK. Update on the management of recurrent Cushing's disease. Neurosurgical Focus. 2015;**38**(2):E16. DOI: 10.3171/2014.11.FOCUS14703

[51] Lindsay JR, Oldfield EH, Stratakis CA, Nieman LK. The postoperative basal cortisol and CRH tests for prediction of long-term remission from Cushing's disease after transsphenoidal surgery. The Journal of Clinical Endocrinology and Metabolism. 2011;**96**(7):2057-2064. DOI: 10.1210/jc.2011-0456

[52] Tritos NA, Biller BM, Swearingen B. Management of Cushing disease. Nature Reviews. Endocrinology. 2011;7(5):279-289. DOI: 10.1038/nrendo.2011.12

[53] Aghi MK. Management of recurrent and refractory Cushing disease. Nature Clinical Practice. Endocrinology & Metabolism. 2008;**4**(10):560-568. DOI: 10.1038/ncpendmet0947

[54] Yamada S, Fukuhara N, Nishioka H, et al. Surgical management and outcomes in patients with Cushing disease with negative pituitary magnetic resonance imaging. World Neurosurgery. 2012;77(3-4):525-532. DOI: 10.1016/j.wneu.2011.06.033

[55] Monteith SJ, Starke RM, Jane JA Jr, Oldfield EH. Use of the histological pseudocapsule in surgery for Cushing disease: Rapid postoperative cortisol decline predicting complete tumor resection. Journal of Neurosurgery. 2012;**116**(4):721-727. DOI: 10.3171/2011.12.JNS11886

[56] Watson JC, Shawker TH, Nieman LK, DeVroom HL, Doppman JL, Oldfield EH. Localization of pituitary adenomas by using

intraoperative ultrasound in patients with Cushing's disease and no demonstrable pituitary tumor on magnetic resonance imaging. Journal of Neurosurgery. 1998;**89**(6):927-932. DOI: 10.3171/jns.1998.89.6.0927

[57] Mayberg M, Reintjes S, Patel A, et al. Dynamics of postoperative serum cortisol after transsphenoidal surgery for Cushing's disease: Implications for immediate reoperation and remission. Journal of Neurosurgery. 2018;**129**(5):1268-1277. DOI: 10.3171/2017.6.JNS17635

[58] Ironside N, Chatain G, Asuzu D, et al. Earlier post-operative hypocortisolemia may predict durable remission from Cushing's disease. European Journal of Endocrinology. 2018;**178**(3):255-263. DOI: 10.1530/EJE-17-0873

[59] Rutkowski MJ, Breshears JD, Kunwar S, Aghi MK, Blevins LS. Approach to the postoperative patient with Cushing's disease. Pituitary. 2015;**18**(2):232-237. DOI: 10.1007/s11102-015-0644-7

[60] Sheehan JP, Xu Z, Salvetti DJ, Schmitt PJ, Vance ML. Results of gamma knife surgery for Cushing's disease. Journal of Neurosurgery. 2013;**119**(6):1486-1492. DOI: 10.3171/2013.7.JNS13217

[61] Mehta GU, Ding D, Patibandla MR, et al. Stereotactic radiosurgery for Cushing disease: Results of an International Multicenter Study. Journal of Clinical Endocrinology and Metabolism. 2017;**102**(11):4284-4291. DOI: 10.1210/jc.2017-01385

[62] Soni P, Koech H, Silva D, et al. Cerebral venous sinus thrombosis after transsphenoidal resection: A rare complication of Cushing disease-associated hypercoagulability. World Neurosurgery. 2020;**134**:86-89. DOI: 10.1016/j.wneu.2019.10.077

[63] Das B, Batool S, Khoja A, Islam N. Presentation, management, and outcomes of nonfunctioning pituitary adenomas: An experience from a developing country. Cureus. 2019;**11**(9):e5759. DOI: 10.7759/cureus.5759

[64] Ntali G, Wass JA. Epidemiology, clinical presentation and diagnosis of non-functioning pituitary adenomas. Pituitary. 2018;**21**(2):111-118. DOI: 10.1007/s11102-018-0869-3

[65] Molitch ME. Pituitary tumours: Pituitary incidentalomas. Best Practice & Research. Clinical Endocrinology & Metabolism. 2009;**23**(5):667-675. DOI: 10.1016/j.beem.2009.05.001

[66] Yavropoulou MP, Tsoli M, Barkas K, Kaltsas G, Grossman A. The natural history and treatment of non-functioning pituitary adenomas (non-functioning PitNETs). Endocrine-Related Cancer. 2020;**27**(10):R375-R390. DOI: 10.1530/ERC-20-0136

[67] Chen L, White WL, Spetzler RF, Xu B. A prospective study of nonfunctioning pituitary adenomas: Presentation, management, and clinical outcome. Journal of Neuro-Oncology. 2011;**102**(1):129-138. DOI: 10.1007/s11060-010-0302-x

[68] Jahangiri A, Wagner JR, Han SW, et al. Improved versus worsened endocrine function after transsphenoidal surgery for nonfunctional pituitary adenomas: Rate, time course, and radiological analysis. Journal of Neurosurgery. 2016;**124**(3):589-595. DOI: 10.3171/2015.1.JNS141543

[69] Freda PU, Bruce JN, Khandji AG, et al. Presenting features in 269 patients with clinically nonfunctioning pituitary adenomas enrolled in a prospective study. Journal of the Endocrine Society. 2020;**4**(4):bvaa021. DOI: 10.1210/jendso/bvaa021

[70] Freda PU, Beckers AM, Katznelson L, et al. Pituitary incidentaloma: An endocrine society clinical practice guideline. The Journal of Clinical Endocrinology and Metabolism. 2011;**96**(4):894-904. DOI: 10.1210/jc.2010-1048

[71] Esposito D, Olsson DS, Ragnarsson O, Buchfelder M, Skoglund T, Johannsson G. Non-functioning pituitary adenomas: Indications for pituitary surgery and post-surgical management. Pituitary. 2019;**22**(4):422-434. DOI: 10.1007/s11102-019-00960-0

[72] Matoušek P, Buzrla P, Reguli Š, Krajča J, Dvořáčková J, Lipina R. Factors that predict the growth of residual nonfunctional pituitary adenomas: Correlations between relapse and cell cycle markers. BioMed Research International. 2018;**2018**:1876290. DOI: 10.1155/2018/1876290

[73] Zada G, Kelly DF, Cohan P, Wang C, Swerdloff R. Endonasal transsphenoidal approach for pituitary adenomas and other sellar lesions: An assessment of efficacy, safety, and patient impressions. Journal of Neurosurgery. 2003;**98**(2):350-358. DOI: 10.3171/jns.2003.98.2.0350

[74] Hadad G, Bassagasteguy L, Carrau RL, et al. A novel reconstructive technique after endoscopic expanded endonasal approaches: Vascular pedicle nasoseptal flap. The Laryngoscope. 2006;**116**(10):1882-1886. DOI: 10.1097/01.mlg.0000234933.37779.e4

[75] Strickland BA, Lucas J, Harris B, et al. Identification and repair of intraoperative cerebrospinal fluid leaks in endonasal transsphenoidal pituitary surgery: Surgical experience in a series of 1002 patients. Journal of Neurosurgery. 2018;**129**(2):425-429. DOI: 10.3171/2017.4.JNS162451

[76] Esquenazi Y, Essayed WI, Singh H, et al. Endoscopic endonasal versus microscopic transsphenoidal surgery for recurrent and/or residual pituitary adenomas. World Neurosurgery. 2017;**101**:186-195. DOI: 10.1016/j.wneu.2017.01.110

[77] Do H, Kshettry VR, Siu A, et al. Extent of resection, visual, and endocrinologic outcomes for endoscopic endonasal surgery for recurrent pituitary adenomas. World Neurosurgery. 2017;**102**:35-41. DOI: 10.1016/j.wneu.2017.02.131

[78] Elshazly K, Kshettry VR, Farrell CJ, Nyquist G, Rosen M, Evans JJ. Clinical outcomes after endoscopic endonasal resection of giant pituitary adenomas. World Neurosurgery. 2018;**114**:e447-e456. DOI: 10.1016/j.wneu.2018.03.006

[79] Jugenburg M, Kovacs K, Stefaneanu L, Scheithauer BW. Vasculature in nontumorous hypophyses, pituitary adenomas, and carcinomas: A quantitative morphologic study. Endocrine Pathology. 1995;**6**(2):115-124. DOI: 10.1007/BF02739874

[80] Borghei-Razavi H, Kshettry VR, Roser F, et al. transcranial surgery for pituitary macroadenomas. In: Quiñones-Hinojosa A, editor. Schmidek and Sweet Operative Neurosurgical Techniques. 7th ed. W.B. Saunders; 2021. pp. 183-193

Section 5

Cavernous Sinus Lesions

Chapter 6

Surgical Approach to the Cavernous Sinus and Middle Cranial, Pterygoid Fossa

Kentaro Watanabe and Sébastien Froelich

Abstract

The cavernous sinus is a very complex area, and surgical treatment requires detailed anatomical knowledge and familiarity with its relationship to surrounding structures. By exposing the lateral wall of the cavernous sinus with the extradural approach, it is possible to pass through the triangular corridor of the cavernous sinus and perform surgical treatment for diseases such as trigeminal schwannoma and meningioma inside and outside the cavernous sinus. In addition to the extradural infratemporal fossa approach, the extradural infratemporal fossa to the pterygoid fossa and the approach to the paranasal sinuses can be safely performed by inserting the endoscope into the bone corridor of the middle cranial fossa. Furthermore, in the last decade, transnasal endoscopic skull based approaches have further developed, facilitating surgical access to the cavernous sinus. The cavernous sinus is an unattachable site due to the complex structure of multiple nerves, veins, and internal carotid arteries, but if the anatomy of the cavernous sinus is known well we can treat this complex site. As for the choice of approach to the cavernous sinus, a better understanding of the anatomy surrounding the cavernous sinus will allow a rational choice between transcranial and transnasal approaches.

Keywords: cavernous sinus, middle fossa approach, endoscopic approach

1. Introduction

This chapter shows the anatomically based bone removal to the original middle cranial fossa surgery method, which is difficult to reach using microscopy alone [1, 2]. The author advocates a safe method of reaching the middle cranial fossa surgery by rationally approaching the cavernous sinus, pterygopalatine fossa, paranasal sinuses from the cranial side, pharynx, and medial jugular foramen from the microanatomical viewpoint [3–5].

In addition, the anatomical relationship with the paranasal sinuses and Eustachian tubes will further enhance the anatomical understanding of transnasal endoscopic surgery. Safe bone removal is paramount in skull base surgery. In this article, it is possible to approach the petrous bone, clivus, sphenoid sinus, maxillary sinus, and ethmoidal sinuses from the infratemporal fossa. Furthermore, understanding the layered structure of the cavernous sinuses will allow for a rational choice of approach to the surgical target and method of tumor removal [6–8].

The various approaches to skull base surgery have a history of significant development through collaboration with pyramidal bone surgery in otolaryngology. As a result, the deepest region, the skull base, can now be safely reached using the pyramidal bone route to the depths of the skull base. Furthermore, since around 2000, neuroendoscopes have been introduced, and transnasal endoscopic surgery has been advocated for the approach through the sphenoid sinus to the sella turcica tumor, the clivus, and the pyramidal bone area [2, 9–13]. In addition, the transcranial approach to reaching surgery has made it possible to use endoscopes to observe deeper regions, expanding the variation of surgery to areas that could not previously be observed with microsurgery. However, despite advances in surgical methods that allow access to the skull base without craniotomy, one of the advantages of nasal endoscopic surgery, it has gradually become clear that endoscopic surgery still has its disadvantages.

Although the surgical wound is not visible in transnasal endoscopic surgery, damage to the mucosa of the nasal cavity can be significant. Because the structures within the nasal cavity have been destroyed, the nasal environment may deteriorate, resulting in nasal contamination, olfactory disturbances, and other symptoms [14].

The most problematic complication is CSF leakage. As safe and reliable methods have been established, the most rational method is selected for each disease based on the direction of tumor extension, site of origin, and surrounding anatomy, craniotomy, endoscopic surgery, and combined approaches of open and endoscopic surgery can be performed safely in response to clinical variations [15–18].

In addition to the conventional middle cranial fossa craniotomy, we have further expanded the range of surgical approaches to the cavernous sinus around the trigeminal nerve by removing bone within a safe range, and by introducing an endoscope, we have expanded the scope of surgical approaches to the cavernous sinus, the inferior cranial nerve, the sinus cavity, and the pterygopalatine fossa. Furthermore, the nasal endoscope was used to approach the cavernous sinus from the pterygopalatine fossa (PPF), and the possibility of treatment from both sides was examined, and the advantages and disadvantages of this approach are discussed.

2. Anatomical structures

2.1 Inferior orbital fissure (IOF)

The IOF is defined as a space between the lateral wall and floor of the orbit. The IOF runs in a direction from the maxillary strut posteriorly to the zygomatic bone anteriorly. The zygomatic nerve (ZyN) of the maxillary nerve, infraorbital nerve (ION), orbital ganglionic branch of PPG, infraorbital artery, and inferior division of ophthalmic vein pass through the IOF [19].

2.2 Muller's muscle (MM)

Muller's muscle, an embryological remnant of the retractor bulbi in mammals, can be identified over the IOF and it blends with the periosteum. Muller's muscle forms a bridge over the IOF, separating the orbital content from the PPF [19].

2.3 Zygomatic nerve (ZyN)

The zygomatic nerve (ZyN) is the first branch of the maxillary nerve that divides off after emerging from the FR to enter the PPF. The ZyN can be found about 5 mm distal from the anterior point of the maxillary strut. Coursing superiorly, it enters the orbit laterally through the IOF. It divides two branches distally, the zygomaticotemporal nerve, which is parasympathetic branch and connected lacrimal nerve, and the zygomaticofacial nerve, which is a sensory branch carried from the skin of the zygomatic area [20].

2.4 Pterygoid fossa

Under the temporalis muscle, the superior head of the lateral pterygoid muscle (LPM) lies on and attaches to the infratemporal surface and infratemporal crest of the greater wing of the sphenoid bone, while the lower head attaches to the lateral surface of the lateral pterygoid plate (LPP). The origin of the Medial pterygoid muscle (MPM) can be seen between the LPP and medial pterygoid plate (MPP). Under the MPP, the wall of epipharynx can be found. The third segment of the internal maxillary artery is located in the pterygoid fossa. The maxillary artery branches into the descending palatine artery, the infraorbital artery, the artery of the pterygoid canal, the artery of the FR, and the sphenopalatine artery [21].

2.5 Vidian nerve

The VN arises from the junction of the greater petrosal nerve and the deep petrosal nerve within the vidian canal, after which it merges with the PPG. Between V2 and V3, the VN lies, on average, 8.0 ± 1,2 mm below V2 and parallel to V2. The bony windows superior and inferior to the VN (between the VN and V2 and between the VN and the superior wall of the pharynx) are the corridor to the posterior SphS [5].

2.6 Sphenoid sinus

The sphenoid sinus is well known as a part of para-sinus which is close to the skull base. It can be used for the transnasal, transsphenoidal approach. However, it can be accessed from the transcranial approach. The posterior part of the SphS can be opened above and below the VN. After exposing and opening the vidian canal, the VN can be followed to the PPG anteriorly. The sphenopalatine artery supplies the SphS mucosa, except for the area of the planum sphenoidal, which is supplied by the posterior ethmoidal artery.

2.7 Maxillary sinus

The posterior wall of the MaxS can be opened below the pterygopalatine fossa through the V2-V3 vidian corridor, between V2 and the palatine nerve. Muller's muscle can be incised along with V2 and the fat around the PPG in the PPF removed. Under V2, the PPG can be translocated medially and inferiorly, thus exposing the upper part of the posterior wall of the MaxS, below the orbit.

3. Extended approaches to the paracavernous sinus

1. Ophthalmo-maxillary nerve corridor (V1-V2 corridor)

2. Maxillary-mandibular corridor (V2-V3 corridor)

3. Extended anterior petrosal approach (petrous rhomboid corridor)

4. Basic exposure of the middle fossa for anterior infratemporal fossa approach

A frontotemporal craniotomy is performed first, with the temporal muscle reflected posteroinferiorly to provide maximal exposure of the anterior temporal base. The pterion and the lesser and greater sphenoid wings are then drilled. The foramen spinosum (FS) and middle meningeal artery (MMA) are identified in the infratemporal fossa extradurally, and the MMA is coagulated and cut. Then, the dura propria is elevated from SOF side or V3 side. The elevation of the dura-propria is performed and exposing SOF, V2, and V3. The lateral wall of the SOF is exposed, and the lateral orbital wall is removed anteriorly exposing the periorbita.

4.1 V1-V2 corridor

sphenoid sinus, maxillary sinus, pterygopalatine fossa (**Figures 1** and 2) [8].

The gap between the ophthalmic and maxillary nerve is used to reach the sphenoid, maxillary, or ethmoid sinuses. This approach is useful when the tumor extends from the periorbital to the infraorbital and further into the middle fossa, with extension into the SphS, MaxS, and PPF. The relationship of the periorbital area to the sinus trigeminal nerve should be known when increasing the tumor removal rate of benign tumors or when performing extensive resection of malignant tumors. Maxillary nerve is exposed along the nerve up to the MaxS. Delete the lateral orbital wall and leading to the middle cranium, the MaxS is covered by the fatty tissue of the PPF. The pterygopalatine ganglion is hidden in the fat tissue within this PPF and the connection between V2 and the vidian nerve can be seen. Initially, the ZyN branches off from the maxillary nerve and heads in the direction of the zygomatic arch. This ZyN is then transected, allowing the PPF to be detached from the orbit. The PPF will be able to deploy V2 backward along with PPG and palatine nerve and vidian nerve.

A large area can be developed between V1-V2. In addition, a small bony ridge at the corner of V1-V2, the Maxillary strut, can be removed just below and anterior to the sphenoid sinus. The infraorbital nerve can be traced peripherally to enter the maxillary sinus. A sphenopalatine artery runs between the sphenoid sinus and the

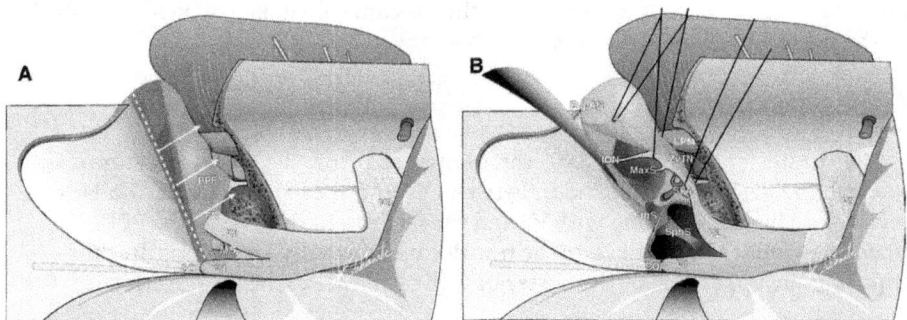

Figure 1.
Schematic images of V1-V2 corridor. A. the V1 and V2 are exposed after removing the bone of the anterior inferior temporal fossa. The PPF, which is included V2 and pterygopalatine ganglion, can be translocated posteriorly. The incision line is shown on the schema. B. after removing the maxillary strut, the sphenoid, ethmoid, and maxillary sinus are opened between the maxillary orbit and pterygopalatine fossa. EthS; ethmoid sinus, FO; foramen ovale, FR; foramen rotundum, ICA; internal carotid artery, ION; inferior orbital nerve, GG: Gasserian ganglion, MaxS; maxillary sinus, PPF: Pterygopalatine fossa, SOF; superior orbital fissure, SPA; sphenopalatine nerve, SphS: Sphenoid sinus, SupAN; superior alveolar nerve, V1; ophthalmic nerve, V2: Maxillary nerve, ZyN; zygomatic nerve.

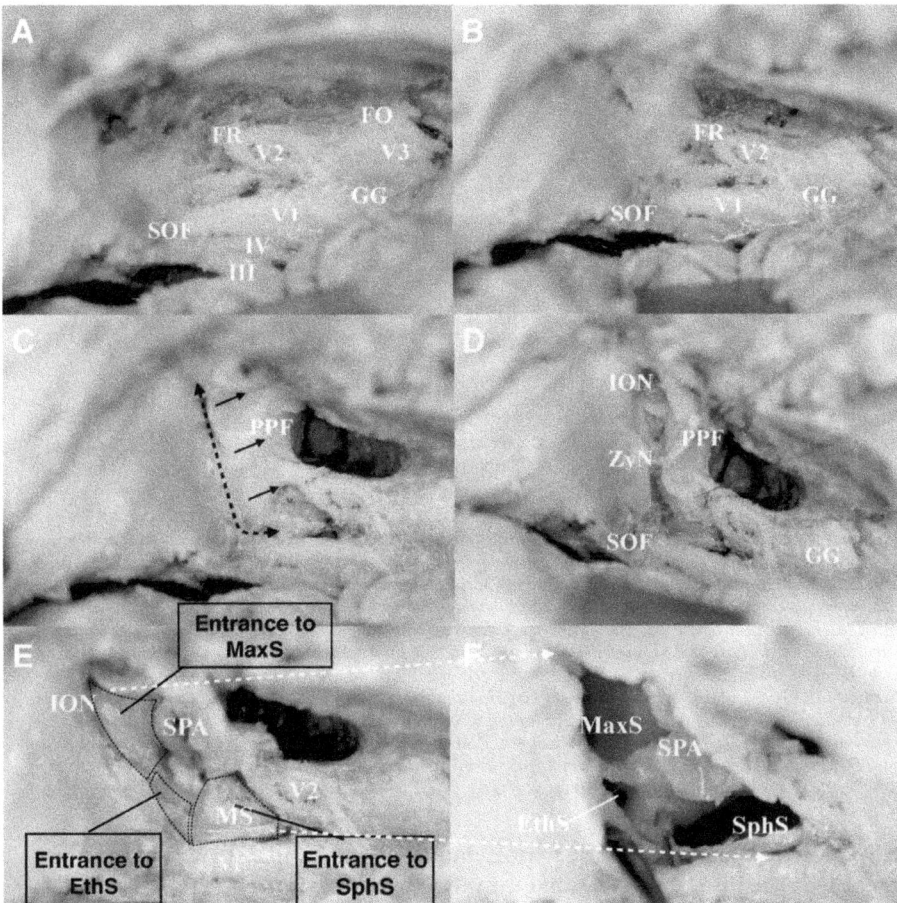

Figure 2.
Stepwise dissections of the anteromedial middle fossa triangle. A. after frontotemporal craniotomy, the middle fossa is exposed with elevation of the dura propria from the cavernous sinus lateral wall. The trigeminal nerve, trochlear nerve, and oculomotor nerve are exposed. B. the lateral orbital wall and orbital roof are removed, and the foramen rotundum is unroofed toward the pterygopalatine fossa. The periorbita and pterygopalatine fossa are exposed. C. an incision is made between the pterygopalatine fossa and orbit. D. the pterygopalatine fossa is translocated posteriorly and the zygomatic nerve is bridged between the pterygopalatine fossa and orbit. E. the bone around the maxillary strut is drilled to get access into the sphenoid sinus. The posterior wall of the maxillary sinus is opened between the maxillary and ophthalmic nerves. F. the maxillary, ethmoid, and sphenoid sinus can be opened through the maxillary and ophthalmic nerves. EthS; ethmoid sinus, FO; foramen ovale, FR; foramen rotundum, ICA; internal carotid artery, ION; inferior orbital nerve, GG: Gasserian ganglion, MaxS; maxillary sinus, PPF; Pterygopalatine fossa, SOF; superior orbital fissure, SPA; sphenopalatine nerve, SphS; Sphenoid sinus, V1; ophthalmic nerve, V2: Maxillary nerve, ZyN; zygomatic nerve.

maxillary sinus, and the exit of the sphenopalatine foramen is visible. This approach is useful for the removal of tumors extending from the anterior middle fossa to the orbital wall, along the trigeminal nerve, or into the maxillary sinus.

4.2 V2-V3 vidian corridor

-sphenoid sinus, maxillary sinus, pterygoid - pharyngeal area, condyle- [6]. Vidian corridor to the para-sinus (**Figure 3**).

The lateral wall of the SOF is exposed, and the lateral orbital wall is removed anteriorly exposing the periorbita. The temporal fossa floor lateral and anterior

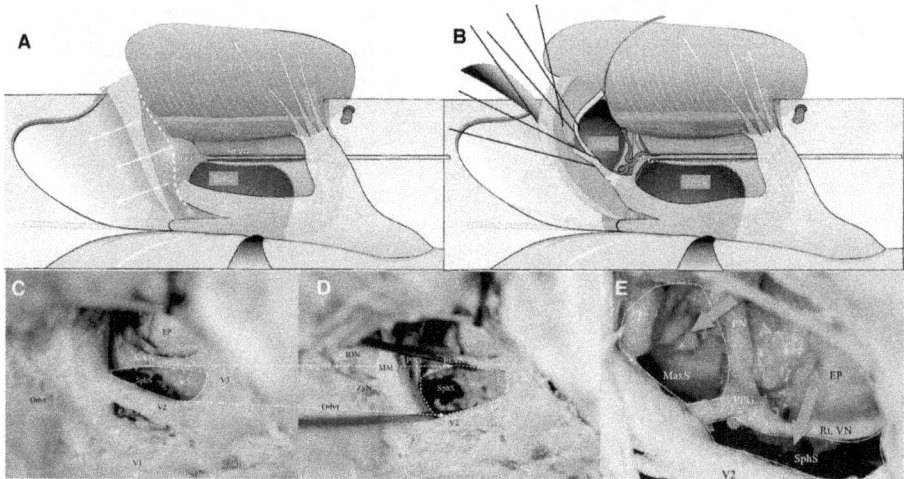

Figure 3.
Schema of the V2-V3 corridor. A. the sphenoid sinus is opened through the vidian corridor. The vidian nerve runs between the V2 and V3, parallel with V2. The sphenoid sinus is opened medially to the vidian nerve. B. the maxillary sinus and sphenoid sinus are opened in the infratemporal fossa with translocation of the fat tissue of the pterygopalatine fossa. The maxillary and sphenoid sinus are opened through the V2-V3 vidian corridor with a lateral corridor of the V2. The blue arrows show the direction of the sinus. C, D, E. the root of pterygoid is drilled and the vidian nerve is exposed completely. The sphenoid sinus can be opened medial to the vidian nerve. Between the vidian nerve and V2, a small corridor can be opened and used to access corridor to the sphenoid sinus. The vidian corridor can be enlarged with retraction of V2 and vidian nerve. EP; epipharynx, EthS; ethmoid sinus, FO; foramen ovale, FR; foramen rotundum, ICA; internal carotid artery, ION; inferior orbital nerve, GG: Gasserian ganglion, MaxS; maxillary sinus, MM; Muller muscle, PPF: Pterygopalatine fossa, SOF; superior orbital fissure, SPA; sphenopalatine nerve, SphS: Sphenoid sinus, V1; ophthalmic nerve, V2: Maxillary nerve, ZyN; zygomatic nerve.

to FO and FR is drilled until the periosteum of the exocranial surface of the bone is reached. The FR is unroofed, and the pterygopalatine fossa is exposed as well as the fascia of the temporalis muscle and lateral pterygoid muscle (LPM). Further elevation of the periosteum of the exocranial surface of the temporal fossa floor can reveal the lateral aspect of the pterygoid process.

Drilling of the antero-superior aspect of the infratemporal fossa, between the LPM and temporal dura mater and lateral orbital wall was done in order to gain additional working space in the pterygoid fossa.

Limits of the pterygoid drilling required are the epipharynx inferiorly, the clivus posteroinferiorly, the posterior wall of the MaxS anteriorly, and the posterior part of the lateral wall of the SphS medially.

Access to the SphS is gained through the V2-V3 vidian corridor, which is in the depth of the FLT and limited superiorly by V2, posteriorly by V3, inferiorly by the superior wall of the pharynx, and anteriorly by the pterygopalatine ganglion (PPG). Following the VN anteriorly, the PPG is identified in the PPF along with the sphenopalatine artery (SPA), which is a branch of the internal maxillary artery (IMA). In some cases, lateral pneumatization of the SphS is extensive and the VN is dehiscent in the SphS. Below V2, the PPF can be opened, and the fat of the PPF removed. This exposes the PPG, SPA, and the posterior wall of the MaxS, which is located between the PPG and the inferior wall of the orbit. Anterior to the PPG and below the orbit, the MaxS can be accessed through this V2-V3 vidian corridor below V2.

The posterior wall of the MaxS is thin and can be opened easily, granting access to a large space to insert the endoscope. At this point, endoscopic assistance is required to provide additional illumination and widen the exposure of the SphS and MaxS.

4.3 Combined V2-V3 corridor and anterior petrosal approach with endoscopic assistance

-Clivus, condyle, dorsal cavernous sinus, medial aspect of the jugular foramen- [7] (**Figure 4**).

The posterior border of the temporal muscle was incised and detached from the temporal bone. The temporal muscle is retracted anteriorly and exposed to the posterior point of the root of zygoma. The temporal craniotomy was performed and access to the middle fossa extradullary.

Initially, the MMA is traced to confirm the foramen spinosum (FS), and the dura mater is thoroughly dissected anteriorly and posteriorly. The arcuate eminence (AE) is identified posteriorly, the GSPN is peeled off posteriorly to expose the pyramidal bone.

The middle meningeal artery (MMA) is coagulated and cut 1 mm out of the FS. The foramen rotundum (FR) is identified anteriorly, where the dura mater enters the bone. An incision is made in the dura above the foramen ovale (FO), and

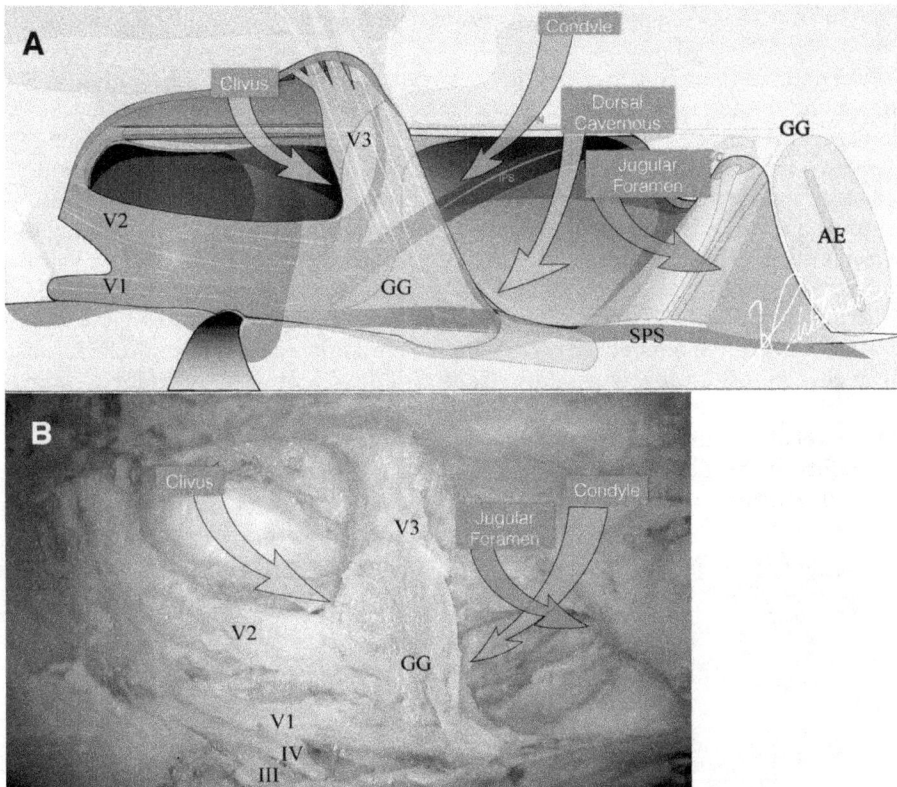

Figure 4.
Schematic representation of the infratemporal fossa, with opening of the vidian corridor and petrous rhomboid. A. the blue arrow shows the direction of access to the upper-mid and lower clivus through the vidian corridor. The green arrow shows the trajectory to the petrous apex and inferior cavernous sinus through the petrous rhomboid. The purple arrow shows the posterior view to the medial jugular foramen and hypoglossal canal through the petrous rhomboid. The light green arrow shows the direction to the clivus. B. the cadaveric view of the middle fossa. The blue arrow shows the direction of access to the upper-mid and lower clivus through the vidian corridor. The purple arrow shows the posterior view of the medial jugular foramen and hypoglossal canal through the petrous rhomboid. The light green arrow shows the direction to the clivus.

one thin layer of dura (osteal dura) is elevated to lift the dura propria and expose the lateral wall of the cavernous sinus [22–26].

After performing the anterior petrosal approach with post meatal drilling, the petrous rhomboid bounded by the GSPN, superior semicircular canal, petrous ridge, and the posterior border of the mandibular verve, gives a working space to the middle and posterior fossa.

The facial, cochlear, and vestibular nerves have a distance from the dura mater of the internal auditory canal (IAC) from this side. Thus, the dura mater can open if they are not compressed and drained by the tumor.

Then, an anterior petrosectomy with extended petrous bone removal toward the petrous apex and ventral cavernous sinus wall through the petrous rhomboid. The bone around the internal auditory canal (IAC) can be removed completely. Usually, the IPS is a landmark of the inferior limit of the anterior petrosal approach.

When the tumor extends to the clivus and/or condyle, the tumor makes a tumor corridor around the petrous and clivus bone. After crossing the IPS, the clivus cancellous bone can be drilled and arrive at the medial aspect of the jugular bulb. A partial clivectomy could be performed by removing bone around the JF.

4.3.1 Anterior view from the petrous rhomboid corridor

The petrous rhomboid area provides a large bone corridor to the petrous and clivus lesion. The endoscopic assistance offers a deep exposure of the middle to lower clivus, epipharyngeal space, and bilateral condylar regions (**Figure 5**). Advancing the petrous rhomboid corridor toward the petrosal apex allows us to drill the bone beneath the Gasserian ganglion. The IPS can be seen where it joins the cavernous sinus. And the ICA is seen rising from the neck just below the GSPN and joining the cavernous sinus. Laterally and anteriorly, the posterior wall of the retropharyngeal mucosa is seen behind the ICA. Care must be taken during exposing the essential structure around the cavernous sinus. Continuing to follow the bony corridor and proceeding with the removal of bone from the clivus, it reaches the mid-clivus until lower clivus. At this time, when the petrous rhomboid and V2-V3 corridor are combined, the posterior aspect of the sphenoid sinus can be reached. Posteroinferiorly, at the level of the mid and lower clivus, it follows to posterior wall of epipharynx. The ability of the V2-V3corridor to provide light assistance and an enlarged working space allows for extra resection of the pterygoid or sphenoid sinus tumor.

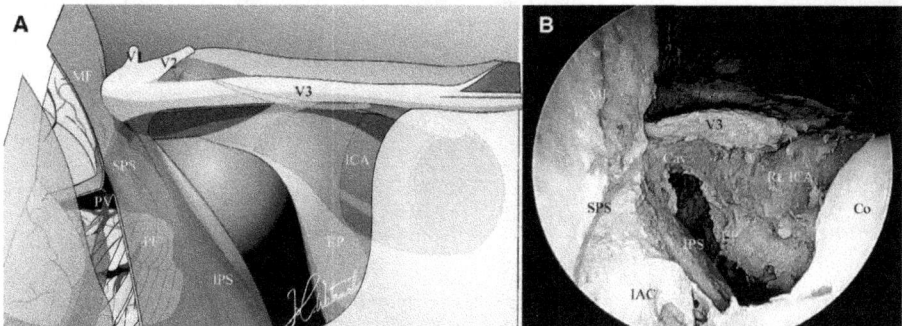

Figure 5.
An endoscopic image and schema and cadaveric dissection image of the anterior view from the anterior petrosal approach. A. an anterior view through the petrous rhomboid corridor after removing the petrous apex and upper clival bone. The ICA goes into the cavernous sinus. The superior and inferior petrosal sinus emerge from the cavernous sinus. B. Below the mandibular nerve (V3), a large cavity can be obtained after removing the petrous apex.

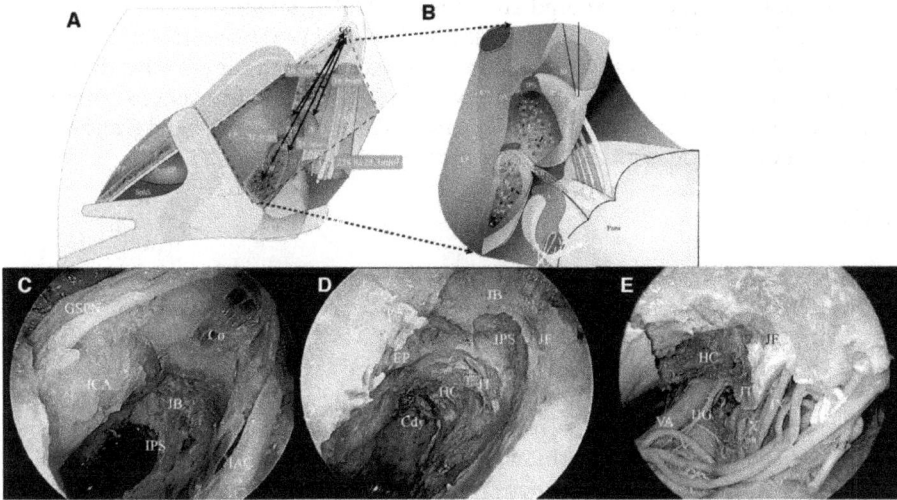

Figure 6.
Posterior view through the petrous rhomboid. A, B. schematic drawing showing a posterior view onto the medial part of the jugular foramen through the petrous rhomboid. C. Endoscopic view, in a posterior trajectory, through the petrous rhomboid. The inferior petrosal sinus, which connects to the medial wall of the jugular bulb, is visualized below the cochlea. D. the horizontal segment of the ICA was skeletonized and followed posteriorly to the vertical segment of the ICA, close to the JB. E. the IPS was cut, exposing the medial wall of the jugular foramen. The jugular tubercle is located between the jugular foramen and hypoglossal canal. Under the hypoglossal canal, the condyle and foramen magnum can be accessed. The dura mater of the posterior fossa was opened. The cranial nerves VII, VIII, IX, X, XI, XII, and vertebral artery can be identified in the intradural space.

4.3.2 Endoscopic-assisted posterior view of the petrous rhomboid to the condyle, medial aspect of the jugular foramen

The IPS leads to finding the location of the medial aspect of the jugular bulb and jugular foramen. To visualize below the IAC, the endoscopic assisted visualization is necessary (**Figure 6**). The posterior view of the petrous rhomboid can provide exposure to the medial jugular complex up to the level of the hypoglossal canal (HGC). The location of the HGC indicates the same level of the condyle. The bone around the condyle is cancellous and can be easily drilled. When the posterior fossa dura is opened, the glossopharyngeal, vagal, and accessory nerves are seen. In the case of tumors originating from the bone, such as chordoma and chondrosarcoma, the tumor provides the surgical corridor by itself. The medial aspect of the jugular bulb is the deepest lesion because of the sigmoid sinus and jugular vein. This route is one of the choices of how to reach the medial jugular lesion.

5. Clinical case

5.1 Case 1

A 58 year old female patient, who operated on 9 years ago for the cavernous sinus meningioma, had an MRI that revealed a recurrence tumor extending into the middle fossa, sphenoid sinus. A pterional approach was performed and exposure of the middle fossa was obtained. An anterior clinoidectomy was performed first. Wide drilling of the bone of the anterior middle fossa was done to remove as much of the tumoral bony infiltration and hyperostosis as possible. The fascia of the pterygoid muscles was exposed and the SOF, Muller muscle, V1 and V2 were skeletonized. A Maxillary strut was drilled and opened the sphenoid sinus between the V1 and V2 corridor. In addition, an incision was made on the posterior border of the Muller's muscle with preserving the zygomatic nerve and transposed anteriorly in order to enlarge the anterior medial triangle. Tumor in the sphenoid sinus was removed under seeing of the endoscope visualization (**Figure 7**).

5.2 Case 2

A 50-year-old male underwent an MRI at a medical health examination. The MRI detected a mass effect in the infratemporal fossa incidentally. The tumor was located in the cavernous sinus and the imaging was evocative of trigeminal schwannoma. The tumor resection was undertaken through a transcranial transcavernous sinus, extradural anterior infratemporal fossa approach. Frontotemporal approach was performed and elevated the frontal and temporal dura from the sphenoid bone. After identifying the superior orbital fissure and elevating the dura propria, the FR and FO were identified and exposed the V1, V2, V3 and the gasserian ganglion. However, the trigeminal nerve fibers lie on the surface of the tumor. In order not to damage the trigeminal nerve fibers, the maxillary strut was drilled and gained the working space to the tumor from the anterior aspect of the tumor. The pterygoid process, between V2 and V3, was thin and was easily drilled to allow wide exposure of the sphenoid sinus. The tumor extension into the SphS was better appreciated under endoscopic visualization. A more extensive resection was accomplished with this approach, although it remained subtotal. The posterior part tumor was removed through the petrous corridor. The pathology was concordant with a schwannoma, from the trigeminal nerve. After tumor resection, the window of

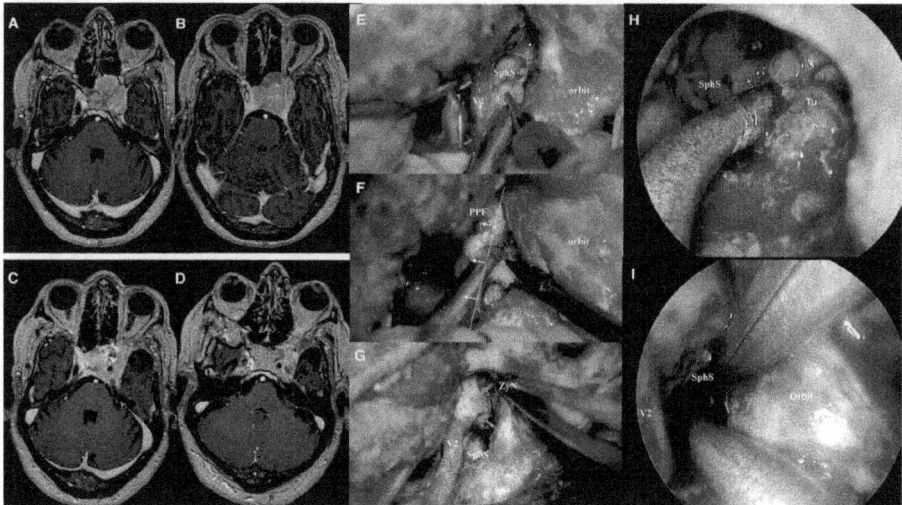

Figure 7.
Pre and post-operation MR images of the cavernous sinus meningioma and intraoperative images of the cavernous meningioma surgery. A, B. preoperative MR image show enhanced mass effect originates from the cavernous sinus extends into the sphenoid sinus. C, D. postoperative MR image shows the yellow arrow showing the removal of the tumor in the sphenoid sinus. E. Sphenoid sinus was opened between the V1 and V2. F. Incision was made between the Muller's muscle and V2. G. the zygomatic temporal nerve was identified in the distal of the V2 and the window of the V1-V2 corridor was enlarged. H. Endoscopic view shows a tumor in the sphenoid sinus and removed with suction. I. Two instruments are inserted through the V1-V2 triangle. IOF; inferior orbital fissure, PPF; pterygopalatine fossa, MM; Muller's muscle, SOF; superior orbital fissure, V1; ophthalmic nerve, V2; maxillary nerve.

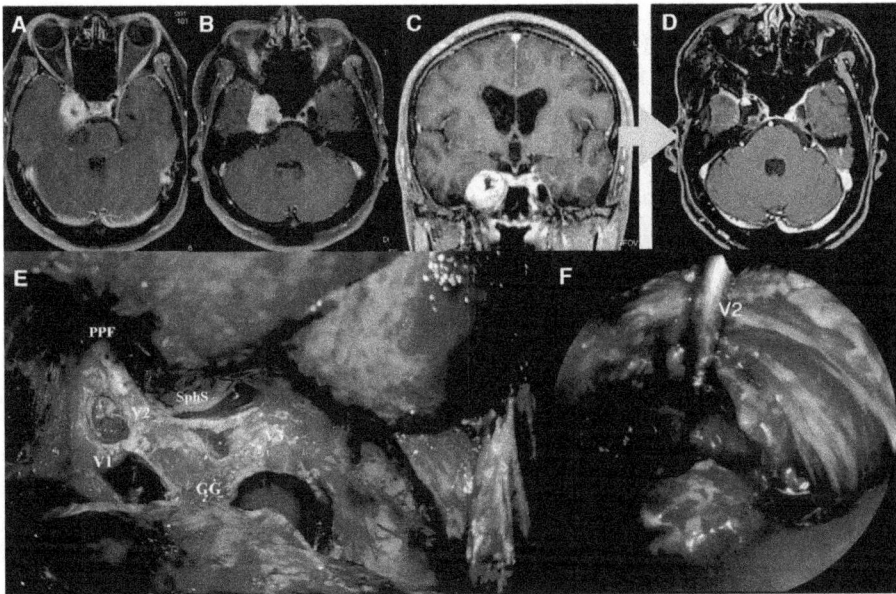

Figure 8.
A: T1 gadolinium enhanced MRI shows a high intensity lesion located in the pterygoid fossa, with an extension up to the sphenoid sinus. B: CT scan shows a mass lesion faces on the sphenoid sinus. C: Post-operative MRI T1 gadolinium image shows the tumor was removed. D; intraoperative microscopic view of the anterior infratemporal fossa view after resection of the tumor. The FLT and AMT were opened, and sphenoid sinus mucosa was seen inside of the sphenoid sinus, between V1-V2 and V2-V3. E; intraoperative endoscopic view below the V2 and the Gasserian ganglion. The tumor can be seen under endoscopic visualization. V1; ophthalmic nerve, V2; maxillary nerve, V3; mandibular nerve, Tu; tumor, SphS; sphenoid sinus, rt.VN; right vidian nerve.

the SphS was covered with a vascularized fascial flap harvested temporal muscle, supplemented by fibrin glue. The postoperative outcome was with slight facial sensation. (**Figure 8A, B, C, D, E**).

Abbreviation

IV	trochlear nerve
III	oculomotor nerve
AE	arcuate eminence
Cdy	condyle
CT	Computed tomography
CTA	computed tomography angiogram
CTV	computed tomography venous angiography
EP	epipharynx
FO	foramen ovale
FR	foramen rotundum
GG	gasserian ganglion
GdT1W	T1 with gadolinium contrast
GSPN	greater superficial petrosal nerve
HC	hypoglossal canal
IAC	Internal auditory canal
ICA	internal carotid
ION	inferior orbital nerve

IPS	inferior petrosal sinus
IJV	internal jugular vein
JB	jugular bulb
JF	Jugular foramen
JT	jugular tubercle
LPM	lateral pterygoid muscle
LPP	lateral pterygoid plate
MPP	medial pterygoid plate
MPM	medial pterygoid muscle
MM	Mullar's muscle
MMA	middle meningeal artery
MF	middle fossa
MRI	magnetic resonance imaging
MS	maxillary strut
PPF	pterygopalatine fossa
PPG	pterygopalatine ganglion
PF	pterygopalatine foramen
SPA	sphenopalatine artery
PLL	petrolingual ligament
ShpS	sphenoid sinus
SOF	superior orbital fissure
SPS	superior petrosal sinus
V1	ophthalmic nerve
V2	maxillary nerve
V3	mandibular nerve
VN	vidian nerve
ZyN	zygomatic nerve

Author details

Kentaro Watanabe[1*] and Sébastien Froelich[2]

1 Department of Neurosurgery, Tokyo Jikei University School of Medicine, Tokyo, Japan

2 Department of Neurorusgery, Hôpital Lariboisière, Paris, France

*Address all correspondence to: k_wtnb0623@jikei.ac.jp

IntechOpen

References

[1] Day JD, Fukushima T, Giannotta SL. Microanatomical study of the extradural middle fossa approach to the petroclival and posterior cavernous sinus region: Description of the rhomboid construct. Neurosurgery. 1994;**34**:1009-1016; discussion 1016

[2] Oyama K, Tahara S, Hirohata T, Ishii Y, Prevedello DM, Carrau RL, et al. Surgical anatomy for the endoscopic Endonasal approach to the ventrolateral Skull Base. Neurologia Medico-Chirurgica (Tokyo). 2017;**57**(10):534-541. DOI: 10.2176/nmc.ra.2017-0039 Epub 2017 Aug 25. PMID: 28845040; PMCID: PMC5638780

[3] Fukushima T, Day JD, Hirahara K. Extradural total petrous apex resection with trigeminal translocation for improved exposure of the posterior cavernous sinus and petroclival region. Skull Base Surgery. 1996;**6**:95-103

[4] Yasuda A, Campero A, Martins C, Rhoton AL Jr, de Oliveira E, Ribas GC. Microsurgical anatomy and approaches to the cavernous sinus. Neurosurgery. 2008;**62**:1240-1263

[5] Ohue S, Fukushima T, Kumon Y, Ohnishi T, Friedman AH. Preauricular transzygomatic anterior infratemporal fossa approach for tumors in or around infratemporal fossa lesions. Neurosurgical Review. 2012;**35**:583-592; discussion 592

[6] Watanabe K, Zomorodi AR, Labidi M, Satoh S, Froelich S, Fukushima T. Visualization of dark side of Skull Base with surgical navigation and endoscopic assistance: Extended petrous rhomboid and rhomboid with maxillary nerve-mandibular nerve Vidian corridor. World Neurosurgery. 2019;**129**:e134-e145. DOI: 10.1016/j. wneu.2019.05.062 Epub 2019 May 17. PMID: 31103769

[7] Watanabe K, Passeri T, Hanakita S, Giammattei L, Zomorodi AR, Fava A, et al. Extradural anterior temporal fossa approach to the paranasal sinuses, nasal cavities through the anterolateral and anteromedial triangles: Combined microscopic and endoscopic strategy. Acta Neurochirurgica. 2021;**163**(8):2165-2175. DOI: 10.1007/s00701-021-04850-y Epub 2021 Apr 29. PMID: 33914166

[8] Oyama K, Watanabe K, Hanakita S, Champagne PO, Passeri T, Voormolen EH, et al. The orbitopterygoid corridor as a deep keyhole for endoscopic access to the paranasal sinuses and clivus. Journal of Neurosurgery. 2020;**134**(5):1480-1489. DOI: 10.3171/2020.3.JNS2022 PMID: 32534497

[9] Kassam A, Snyderman CH, Mintz A, Gardner P, Carrau RL. Expanded endonasal approach: The rostrocaudal axis. Part I. Crista galli to the Sella turcica. Neurosurgical Focus. 2005;**19**(1):E3 PMID: 16078817

[10] Kassam A, Snyderman CH, Mintz A, Gardner P, Carrau RL. Expanded endonasal approach: The rostrocaudal axis. Part II. Posterior clinoids to the foramen magnum. Neurosurgical Focus. 2005;**19**(1):E4 PMID: 16078818

[11] Kassam AB, Vescan AD, Carrau RL, Prevedello DM, Gardner P, Mintz AH, et al. Expanded endonasal approach: Vidian canal as a landmark to the petrous internal carotid artery. Journal of Neurosurgery. 2008;**108**(1):177-183. DOI: 10.3171/JNS/2008/108/01/0177 PMID: 18173330

[12] Hanakita S, Chang WC, Watanabe K, Ronconi D, Labidi M, Park HH, et al. Endoscopic Endonasal approach to the anteromedial temporal fossa and mobilization of the Lateral Wall of the cavernous sinus through the

inferior orbital fissure and V1-V2 corridor: An anatomic study and clinical considerations. World Neurosurgery. 2018;**116**:e169-e178. DOI: 10.1016/j.wneu.2018.04.146 Epub 2018 Apr 27. PMID: 29709753

[13] Mehta GU, Raza SM. Endoscopic endonasal transpterygoid approach to petrous pathologies: Technique, limitations and alternative approaches. Journal of Neurosurgical Sciences. 2018;**62**(3):339-346. DOI: 10.23736/S0390-5616.18.04302-3 Epub 2018 Jan 10. PMID: 29327863

[14] Kuan EC, Suh JD, Wang MB. Empty nose syndrome. Current Allergy and Asthma Reports. 2015;**15**(1):493. DOI: 10.1007/s11882-014-0493-x PMID: 25430954

[15] Martin TJ, Loehrl TA. Endoscopic CSF leak repair. Current Opinion in Otolaryngology & Head and Neck Surgery. 2007;**15**(1):35-39. DOI: 10.1097/MOO.0b013e3280123fce PMID: 17211181

[16] Hannan CJ, Almhanedi H, Al-Mahfoudh R, Bhojak M, Looby S, Javadpour M. Predicting post-operative cerebrospinal fluid (CSF) leak following endoscopic transnasal pituitary and anterior skull base surgery: A multivariate analysis. Acta Neurochirurgica. 2020;**162**(6):1309-1315. DOI: 10.1007/s00701-020-04334-5 Epub 2020 Apr 21. PMID: 32318930

[17] Algattas H, Setty P, Goldschmidt E, Wang EW, Tyler-Kabara EC, Snyderman CH, et al. Endoscopic Endonasal approach for Craniopharyngiomas with intraventricular extension: Case series, long-term outcomes, and review. World Neurosurgery. 2020;**144**:e447-e459. DOI: 10.1016/j.wneu.2020.08.184 Epub 2020 Sep 2. PMID: 32890848

[18] Ishii Y, Tahara S, Hattori Y, Teramoto A, Morita A, Matsuno A. Fascia patchwork closure for endoscopic endonasal skull base surgery. Neurosurgical Review. 2015;**38**(3):551-556. DOI: 10.1007/s10143-015-0614-6 discussion 556-7Epub 2015 Feb 14. PMID: 25675847

[19] De Battista JC, Zimmer LA, Rodríguez-Vázquez JF, Froelich SC, Theodosopoulos PV, DePowell JJ, et al. Muller's muscle, no longer vestigial in endoscopic surgery. World Neurosurgery. 2011;**76**(3-4):342-346. DOI: 10.1016/j.wneu.2010.12.057 PMID: 21986434

[20] Khalid S, Iwanaga J, Loukas M, Tubbs RS. Bilateral absence of the zygomatic nerve and Zygomaticofacial nerve and foramina. Cureus. 2017;**9**(7):e1505. DOI: 10.7759/cureus.1505 PMID: 28948125; PMCID: PMC5608499

[21] Alokby G, Albathi A, Alshurafa Z, AlQahtani A. Endoscopic endonasal repair of a temporal lobe meningoencephalocele in the pterygoid fossa: A case report and literature review. International Journal of Surgery Case Reports. 2021;**83**:105963. DOI: 10.1016/j.ijscr.2021.105963 Epub 2021 May 12. PMID: 34022760; PMCID: PMC8164042

[22] Goel A. Extended middle fossa approach for petroclival lesions. Acta Neurochirurgica. 1995;**135**:78-83

[23] Kawase T, Shiobara R, Toya S. Anterior transpetrosal-transtentorial approach for sphenopetroclival meningiomas: Surgical method and results in 10 patients. Neurosurgery. 1991;**28**:869-875; discussion 875-866

[24] Kawase T, Shiobara R, Toya S. Middle fossa transpetrosal-transtentorial approaches for petroclival meningiomas. Selective pyramid resection and radicality. Acta Neurochirurgica. 1994;**129**:113-120

[25] Kawase T, Toya S, Shiobara R, Mine T. Transpetrosal approach for

aneurysms of the lower basilar artery.
Journal of Neurosurgery.
1985;**63**:857-861

[26] Borghei-Razavi H, Tomio R,
Fereshtehnejad SM, Shibao S, Schick U,
Toda M, et al. Anterior petrosal
approach: The safety of Kawase triangle
as an anatomical landmark for anterior
petrosectomy in petroclival
meningiomas. Clinical Neurology and
Neurosurgery. 2015;**139**:282-287

Section 6

Chordomas

Chapter 7

Challenges in Diagnosing Chordoma (Skull Base Tumors)

Amit Kumar Chowhan and Pavan Kumar G. Kale

Abstract

Chordoma is a rare bone malignancy that influences the spine and cranium base. Once in a while, it includes bone and when it does, cranial bones are the favored location. Chordomas emerge from embryonic remnants of the primitive notochord and chondrosarcomas from primitive mesenchymal cells, otherwise from the embryonic rest of the cranial cartilaginous matrix. Chondrosarcomas constitute a heterogeneous group of essential bone malignancy characterized by hyaline cartilaginous neoplastic tissue. Both are characterized by invasion and pulverization of the neighboring bone and delicate tissue with higher locoregional reappearance frequency. Chordoma and chondrosarcoma, especially myxoid variation of chondrosarcoma of the cranium base, are as often as possible amalgamated because of similar anatomic location, clinical presentation, and radiologic sightings, and mixed up histopathological highlights. Chordoma and chondrosarcoma vary with respect to their origin, management strategy, and contrast particularly with respect to outcome. Ultimately, developing indication supports aberrant growth factor signaling as possible pathogenic mechanisms in chordoma. Here, we have shown such a location-based symptomatic predicament, understood effectively with ancillary immunohistochemistry. In this review, we summarize the most recent research findings and focus primarily on the pathophysiology and diagnostic aspects.

Keywords: chordoma, chondrosarcoma, histopathology, immunohistochemistry, spheno-occiput

1. Introduction

Chordomas are uncommon, locally aggressive malignant bone tumors that develop from the primordial notochord remnants, accounting for 1–4% of all primary malignant bone tumors [1]. Despite the fact that they can form anywhere along the axial skeleton, sacrococcygeal and spheno-occipital locations are most prevalent, followed by cervicothoracic and coccyx [2]. There are also reports of axial destinations and soft tissue involvement. The spheno-occipital synchondrosis of the clivus is the most common source of intracranial chordomas. The origin can be found along the upper clivus (basisphenoid) or along the clivus' caudal border (basiocciput). Intracranial chordomas can sometimes develop singly from the petrous apex. Chordomas are classified into three categories based on their histological characteristics: classical (conventional), chondroid, and dedifferentiated. Chondroid chordoma is a relatively rare variant that accounts for nearly 14% of all chordomas and is thought to have a better prognosis than classical chordoma [3].

Dedifferentiated chondrosarcoma is a type of cartilaginous tumor that includes two distinct components, namely low-grade chondrogenic components and high-grade noncartilaginous sarcoma. It constitutes 1–2% of all primary bone tumors. Dedifferentiated chondrosarcoma is a rare, highly malignant variant of chondrosarcoma and has a poor prognosis.

Chondrosarcoma is the collective term for a group of heterogeneous, premalignant tumors of bone characterized by the arrangement of hyaline cartilaginous neoplastic tissue. Most conventional chondrosarcomas are low- to intermediate-grade tumors (grade 1 or grade 2). Dedifferentiated chondrosarcoma develops when low-grade conventional chondrosarcoma changes into a high-grade sarcoma, most often showing features of osteosarcoma, fibrosarcoma, or else undifferentiated pleomorphic sarcoma. Mesenchymal Chondrosarcoma (MCS) could be a profoundly malignant tumor showing a Dimorphic histologic design with an exceedingly undifferentiated round cell component admixed with well-differentiated cartilage. The myxoid variant of chondrosarcoma is usually seen in soft tissues, identified as Chordoid sarcoma or parachordoma [4]. Seldom, it includes bone and when it does, cranial bones are the favored location. The prognosis for the majority of patients with chondrosarcoma is relatively favorable and relates to histologic evaluation and satisfactory surgical margins.

In any case, the complex anatomy of the spine and generally expansive tumor volume makes a clean resection ideally challenging, driving to a higher proportion of local relapse as well as distant metastases. Latest disclosures in molecular biology and epigenetics of chordoma and chondrosarcomas have significantly advanced our understanding of the pathobiology of these tumors and offer insight into potential restorative targets.

2. History

The first macroscopical and microscopical description of chordomas was given by the German pathologist Rudolf Virchow and depicted on autopsy an incidental, little, slimy development on the surface of clivus [5]. Virchow coined the term "chordomata", and he described its embryonic character and denoted it as 'ecchondrosisphysaliforaspheno-occipitalis' which translates to a "cartilaginous physaliphorous" lesion of the cartilaginous junction between basiocciptal and basisphenoid bones [6]. He used the word "physaliphora" to describe the findings during his microscopic observations. Hugo Ribbert, another German pathologist afterwards proposed the term chordoma.

In 1858, German anatomist Johannes Peter Müller hypothesized that chordomata may originate from notochordal tissue. Müller's hypothesis was based on the point that most vertebrates, counting humans, contain remnants of notochordal tissues but his hypothesis was rejected by Virchow and Luschka (A German anatomist and one of the most prolific anatomical writers of the 19th century) due to a lack of evidence. After a few years later Belgian anatomist Hector Leboucq proposed that notochordal tissue is demolished before human birth [7]. Arnold C. Klebs, a Swiss physician in 1864 first described a patient with spheno-occipital chordomata and afterward in 1889, he stated the first case of cervical vertebrae chordomata. In 1910, physicians Feldmann and Mazzia reported the first official case of a sacrococcygeal Chordoma. In 1919, physician Daland in the USA operated on the first spheno-occipital case. In this year Porter and Daland attempted X-ray treatments on their patient. In 1960, Hungarian neurosurgeons Zoltan and Fenyes noted various initial operation cases to treat cranial chordomas.

3. Epidemiology

Cranium base chordomas are unusual malignancies with an incidence rate of less than 0.2% among all intracranial neoplasms [8]. Population-based studies also confirmed that the overall frequency of chordomas in a year to be 0.08 per 100,000 persons [8]. All age groups have the chance to be affected with this disease but most of the cases are diagnosed during adulthood and hardly affect children and adolescents. Approximately 0.15% of all intracranial neoplasms are detected as Chondrosarcomas and it is 6% of all cranium base tumors [8].

4. Pathogenesis

4.1 Origin

In general, it is believed that chordoma cells are initiated from the embryonic notochord remnants [9]. It is also projected that notochordal remnants are derived from the embryonic notochord and reside in the region of an embryo where the embryonic notochord was existing. It is assumed that notochordal remnants stay dormant in maximum cases but might be transformed into malignancies. Yamaguchi and his colleagues have stated a link between persistent notochordal remnants and Chordoma [10]. Currently, cancer stem cell theory has given more details about the embryonic transformations and stem-like cells in Chordoma may show stemness, gene expression, and differentiation [9].

Chordomas may also be an outcome of direct malignant transformation of the notochordal remnant, deprived of a benign notochordal tumor intermediary stage. Otherwise chordoma may be inferred from benign notochordal cell tumor through malignant transformation (**Figure 1**) making another root of chordomagenesis.

4.2 Chromosome

Chromosomal changes are found in a few *de novo* chordomas having poorer prognosis and most common genomic alterations are observed in chromosome numbers 1p, 3, 4, 9, 10, 13, and 14 [11]. It was found that chromosomal gain is less common than chromosomal deletion. Bai and his colleagues have identified

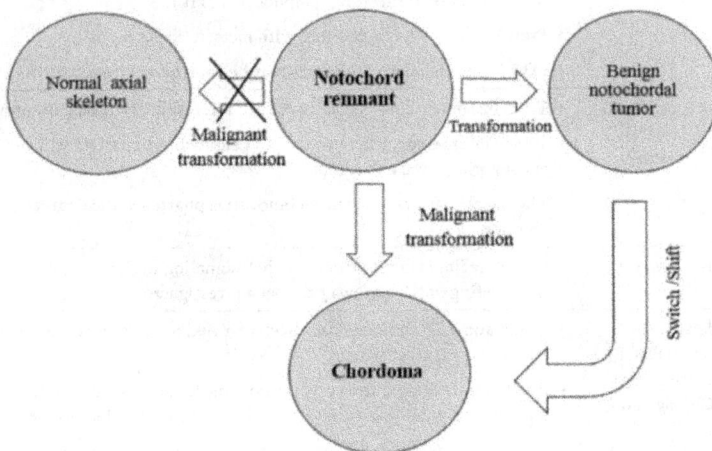

Figure 1.
A schematic presentation of notochord remnant and Chordoma [9].

Approach	Description
Brachyury	• Expression of this protein is the diagnostic hallmark of chordoma.
	• Encoded by T-Box Transcription Factor T (TBXT) or T gene
	• Germline duplications of the T gene are associated with familial chordomas, whereas somatic tandem T duplications are related with sporadic chordoma.
	• Brachyury is a mediator of epithelial-to-mesenchymal transition by down-regulating E-cadherin expression.
	• Ubiquitous brachyury expression in chordoma makes this protein a therapeutic target.
Cyclin-dependent kinase inhibitor 2A (CDKN2A)	• Upregulation of other T-box genes in malignancy is supposed to repress cell-cycle regulators such as CDKN2A.
	• Tumor suppressor proteins are also encoded by the CDKN2A gene.
	• Mutations of the CDKN2A gene results in uncontrolled cell proliferation through activation of cyclin-dependent kinases 4 and 6 (CDK4/6).
Phosphate and tensin homolog (PTEN)	• PTEN gene encodes for a tumor suppressor protein.
	• PTEN is a potent cell growth regulator.
	• Numerous chordomas feature loss of PTEN function whereas up-regulation of PTEN has been investigated.
Chromatin Remodeling	• Pathogenesis of chordoma may involve dysregulation in DNA level resulting in oncogene activation or tumor suppressor silencing.
	• Mutations of Switch/Sucrose non-fermentable (SWI/SNF) gene results in chromatin dysregulation, assisting neoplastic development.
	• SMARCB1 gene is a SWI/SNF component that is supposed to act as tumor suppressor by regulating histone methylation of transcription factor EZH2.
	• Loss of SMARCB1 function acts as a defining marker of poorly differentiated chordomas.
	• Mutations in other SWI/SNF associates like PBRM1, SETD2, ARID1A, etc. have been recognized as probable drivers in chordomas.
Immune Checkpoint: Programmed cell death protein 1/ Programmed Cell Death Ligand 1 (PD-1/ PD-L1)	• Recent immunotherapy trials of chordoma have focused on immune checkpoint regulator, PD-L1, which is responsible for suppressing regulatory T cell apoptosis.
	• PD-L1 expression is also observed on lymphocytes and tumor-infiltrating macrophages at the tumor-stroma interface.
	• Chordomas with negative PDL1 expression is inclined to have further PD-L1 positive tumor-infiltrating lymphocytes (TIL).
	• Prevalence of TIL is associated with metastatic potential.
	• PD-L1 expression in chordomas may be controlled by microRNAs.
T-cell immunoglobulin and mucin-domain 3 (TIM3)/ galectin-9 (Gal9)	• TIM3 has newly emerged as a target of interest in chordoma immunotherapy.
	• TIM3 endorses survival of the tumor cells by binding to galectin-9 (Gal9) and encouraging T cell exhaustion.
	• TIM3/Gal9 pathway may be an innovative pharmaceutical target for chordoma.
Hedgehog pathway	• Given the important role of hedgehog signaling in chondrogenesis, therapeutic targeting of this pathway has been investigated.
Platelet-derived growth factor (PDGF) and epidermal growth factor (EGF) signaling Pathways	• PDGF and EGF signaling have been revealed to increase tumor hyperplasia and tumor survival also.
	• PDGF and EGF bind to a receptor tyrosine kinase resulting in the initiation of regulatory signaling pathways of proliferation and differentiation.
	• Tyrosine kinase inhibitors can selectively block PDGF and EGF receptors phosphorylation and this can be applied for the treatment of chordoma.

Approach	Description
PI3K/Akt/mTOR Pathway	• Phosphoinositide 3-kinase (PI3K)/Akt signaling pathway regulates progression of the cell cycle, cellular proliferation, and survival.
	• Mutations in mTOR and tumor suppressors of PI3K/Akt cascade have been connected with oncogenesis.
	• Skull-based chordoma cells with higher brachyury expression show upregulation of PI3K/AKT cascade genes compared to low-brachyury tumor cells.
	• PI3K/AKT pathway inhibitors decrease brachyury expression.
Insulin-like growth factor 1 (IGF-1) Pathway	• IGF-1 affects mitogenic activity in bone and its dysregulation may accelerate chordoma development.
	• IGF-1/IGF-1 receptor expression and prognosis in chordomas have been reported.
	• Activation of IGF-1 receptor signaling can thus contribute to the progression of chordoma cells, denoting as a potential biomarker.
Collagen Type II Alpha 1 Chain (COL2A1)	• *COL2A1* codes α-chain of type II collagen fibers, a key collagen component of articular cartilage.
	• COL2A1 mutations may generate vital perturbation of matrix deposition and oncogenic signaling of chondrosarcoma.
Extracellular matrix	• Chordomas produce a plentiful extracellular matrix.
	• Cathepsin K, a cysteine protease may play a role in osteoclast-mediated bone resorption.
	• There is a relation between the expression of cathepsin K and chordoma.
	• Morphogens, signaling molecules that govern embryonic notochord development may play a key role to establish a cellular microenvironment that stimulates chordoma pathogenesis.
MicroRNA (miRNAs)	• miRNAs are involved in normal chondrogenesis like miR-140 negatively regulates histone deacetylase 4 in non-hypertrophic chondrocytes.
	• Histone deacetylase 4 regulates the chondrocyte hypertrophic phase by inhibiting transcription factor RUNX2 (Runt-related transcription factor 2).
Hypoxia-inducible factor-1α (HIF-1α)	• Expression of the pro-angiogenic ligand vascular endothelial growth factor (VEGF) is dependent upon HIF-1α.
	• HIF-1α is upregulated under hypoxic environments.
	• During hypoxia, normal and malignant chondrocytes induce HIF-1α expression.
Other molecular targets	• Phosphatidylinositol-4,5-Bisphosphate 3-Kinase catalytic subunit Alpha (PIK3CA) mutations are key aspects of chordoma pathogenesis and therefore it is a potential target.
	• Receptor tyrosine kinases (RTKs) are the key players in the development and progression of chordoma.
	• Human epidermal growth factor receptor 2 (HER2)/neu is associated with EGF receptor dimer formation.
	• There is a possibility that this heterodimerization upsurges the sensitivity of EGFR-positive chordoma.

Table 1.
Different pathways and cyto-molecular factors associated with the pathogenesis of Chordoma [11, 13, 14].

germline duplication of the TBXT gene that encodes brachyury, a transcription factor that plays an important role in familial Chordoma [12]. A common genetic polymorphism in *TBXT* is consequently associated with an increased risk for both sporadic and familial chordoma. They have found that *PBRM1, B2M* and *MAP3K4* are the most frequently mutated cancer driver genes in chordoma. Given the role of *PBRM1* and *SETD2* in chromatin remodeling, it can be proposed that epigenetic dysregulation may play a vital role in chordoma development. Bai and his group suggested that amplifications of *TBXT* gene, homozygous deletion of *CDKN2A* and mutations in genes like *PBRM1*, *SETD2*, *ARID1A* etc. are the most common genomic events in sacral Chordoma [12].

4.3 Different pathways

Developing new technologies have widened our understanding of chordoma by implicating innovative pathways to understand the pathogenesis and future therapeutic approach. Alteration in cell-cycle regulation and different signaling pathways have been identified in chordomas. It is also well established that different growth factor signaling is also related to pathogenic mechanisms in chordoma. There are a number of pathways and cyto-molecular factors which are associated with the pathogenesis of chordoma and some are listed in **Table 1**.

4.4 Epigenetics

Critically, myxoid chondrosarcoma harbors repetitive genetic rearrangements including the NR4A3 gene, demonstrating an exceptionally useful confirmatory diagnostic indication. Other proteins namely EWSR1 and TAF15 are also involved in this type of cancer. Some researchers also described uncommon combination of transcripts like HSPA8-NR4A3, TFG-NR4A3, and TCF12-NR4A3 which can play a major role in the initiation and development of this malignancy [15]. Currently, no predictive factor is accessible to assist decision making for this metastatic process, and in specific to characterize whether systemic treatment ought to be utilized.

5. Clinical presentation

Patients with chordomas and chondrosarcomas generally show common and occasionally confusing symptoms, which sometimes delay the diagnosis process until the late stages of the illness [16]. Presentation of the tumors can essentially shift depending on the area of the tumor, expansion, and vicinity of the lesion to basic structures. Visual indications may incorporate obscured vision or loss of vision, ptosis, and visual field defects related to cranial nerve palsies that may be clarified by the area and development pattern of the tumors. It is common for chordoma to invade structures such as petroclival region, parapharyngeal space, cavernous sinus, temporal bone, cerebellopontine point, and infratemporal fossa. Headache, seizures, weakness, vomiting, etc. are the most common symptom in the case of chordoma.

Sacrococcygeal chordoma has different symptomatology based on the location. Most patients usually present with a posterior sacral mass initially and in later stages present with features of sacral pain, lower limb weakness, and/or bladder bowel disturbances.

Other signs and side effects that will show with clival lesions are hypoesthesia, hearing loss, dysphonia, vertigo, dysphagia, dysarthria, dyspnea, and anosmia. Bigger size/volume tumors may likewise compress the brainstem and cerebellum, affecting ataxia, gait disturbances, dysmetria, hemiparesis, or tetraparesis [17]. It is very tough to recognize the nature of the tumor on the basis of the only clinical demonstration. Basic similarities, differences, and treatment difficulties are shown in **Table 2**.

General features	Chordomas and Chondrosarcomas
Similarity	• Chordoma and chondrosarcoma of the skull base are rare tumors with overlapping presentations and anatomic locations. Chordomas, mostly occur at the sacrococcygeal region, and at the sphen-occipital region, with nearly all of these occurring at the clivus. Chordoma and chondrosarcoma constitute most primary bone tumors arising within the skull base, both are characterized by invasion and pulverization of the neighboring bone and delicate tissue with higher locoregional reappearance frequency.
	• All age groups have the chance to be affected but most of the cases are diagnosed during adulthood and hardly affect children and adolescents. These diseases affect males more often than females.
	• Chordoma and chondrosarcoma have an alike radiologic and histologic appearance.
	• Display slow growth patterns and cause gradual displacement of neurovascular structures, in sequence leading to the expression of clinical signs and subsequent diagnosis.
	• High tendency for locoregional recurrence with infiltration and obliteration of the surrounding bone and soft tissue.
	• Metastatic potential is considered to be relatively low, distant metastases have been described in patients with advanced disease.
	• Poor prognosis and a lesser survival rate.
Differences	• Chordomas arise from embryonic remnants of the primitive notochord with a molecular alteration preceding their malignant transformation. Chondrosarcomas originate from primitive mesenchymal cells or from embryonic remnants of the cartilaginous matrix in the cranium.
	• MRI characteristics in *de novo* cases of chordoma, chondroid chordoma, and chondrosarcoma have shown some differences. Most of the chordomas are located in the midline craniovertebral axis whereas in cases of chondrosarcoma the preferred location is paramedian adjacent to synchondrosis [18, 19].
	• Light microscopic examination shows that most chordomas from the base of the skull and spine had classic features. It consists of sheets, nests, and cords of large cohesive cells in a myxoid matrix. Maximum chondrosarcomas are of mixed hyaline and myxoid type and they differ from chordoma by their cytologic and architectural features.
Challenges	• The multifaceted structure of the cranial base, composed with the close proximity to cranial nerves and vessels, signifies a weighty challenge in the management of these tumors.
	• Aggressive surgery is associated with a considerable risk of high morbidity and mortality and in case of partial resection locoregional recurrence is the rule. Most patients require some kind of adjuvant therapy for disease control.

Table 2.
Similarities, differences, and treatment difficulties of both chordomas and chondrosarcomas.

6. Diagnosis

Chordoma and chondrosarcoma have a common overview and similar anatomic location, and can be troublesome to recognize some time before the histopathologic and immunohistochemical examination; in any case, tumors have a distinctive origin and distinctive prognosis. Chondroid chordomas, in spite of having a few pathologic characteristics that are comparable to chondrosarcoma, carry on clinically like chordomas. The preoperative separation between chordomas and chondrosarcomas based on the clinical presentation and clinical and instrument-based diagnostics alone is very tough.

Intracranial chordomas usually have a midline cranium base area whereas most chondrosarcomas emerge along the petro-occipital fissure. On the other hand, chondrosarcomas may sometimes have a midline area, making it difficult to differentiate between chondrosarcoma and an intracranial chordoma. In addition, these two tumors have alike signal intensity on T1- and T2-weighted magnetic resonance images. Hence, direct, globular, or arc-like calcifications when present in chondrosarcomas may help to distinguish them from intracranial chordomas [20].

Plasmacytoma and lymphoma sometimes include the cranium base and cause damage to lytic bone. Craniopharyngiomas, other than illustrating a generally characteristic signal intensity, are found more anteriorly in midline than are intracranial chordomas. Other differentials, though uncommon, may include aggressive pituitary adenoma, histiocytosis X, trigeminal neuroma, dermoid and epidermoid cyst.

Neurosurgical methods frequently utilized for the resection of intracranial chordomas and chondrosarcomas are trans-sphenoidal, Cranio-orbito-zygomatic, transbasal, transcondylar, transzygomatic amplified center fossa, and transmaxillary methodologies. Chordomas and chondrosarcomas are not sensitive to chemotherapy and thus the management modality might be a combination of surgical resection with a maximal extraction and adjuvant radiotherapy for both chondrosarcomas and chordomas.

Differential diagnosis includes mainly metastatic carcinoma, chondrosarcoma, and myxopapillary ependymoma. Metastatic carcinoma and chordomas both show positive responses with epithelial markers. It is unusual for metastatic carcinoma to have the lobulated growth pattern of chordoma whereas chondrosarcoma may grow in a lobulated pattern but without fibrous septa. Myxopapillary ependymoma is easy to differentiate from chordoma as they do not stain for epithelial markers [21]. In electron, microscopic view chordoma shows desmosome and mitochondrial rough endoplasmic reticulum complex whereas both are absent in case of chondrosarcoma [22].

6.1 Radiology

Cranium base chordomas are ordinarily found within the midline [18] and appear to start within the bone, penetrating the way of slightest resistance and inevitably creating a soft tissue mass. In spite of the fact that their clinical and imaging presentations are analogous, they infer from distinctive roots. CT and MRI, both are required for accurate characterization of clival chordomas and their association to adjacent anatomy (**Figures 2** and **3**). Currently, MRI is the most suitable for the radiologic evaluation of intracranial chordomas [23].

Chowhan and his colleagues (2012) studied through MRI of chondrosarcoma and showed a T2 hyperintense lesion involving the clivus, petrous temporal bone, and sphenoid bone [4]. This lesion was hypointense on a T1-weighted image (**Figure 4a**) and enhanced heterogeneously in the postcontrast (gadolinium) study (**Figure 4b**).

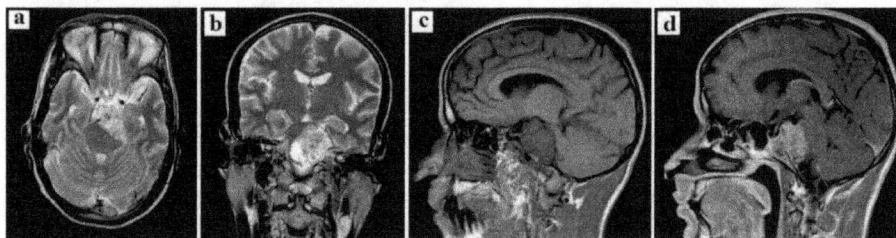

Figure 2.
MRI: *Expansile lobulated lytic lesion in clivus which is hyperintense on T2 images (a, b) hypointense on T1 (c) image showing heterogeneous enhancement after contrast administration (d) extending into cisterns causing compression over brainstem and displacing basilar artery, lesion is extending into sella (red arrow).*

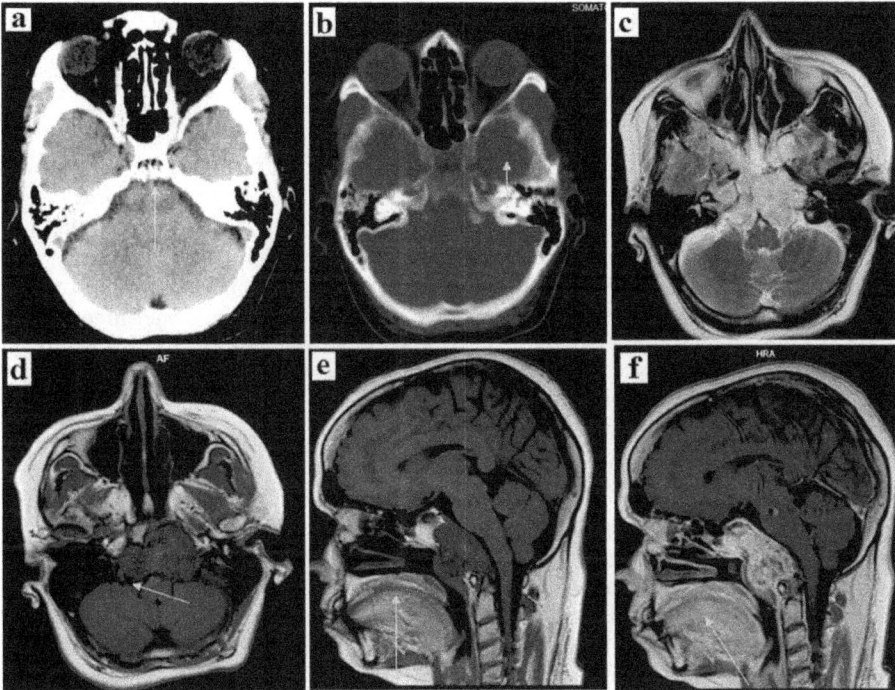

Figure 3.
Figure (a) axial CT brain window and figure (b) axial CT bone window showing subtle lesion on brain window and small lytic lesion on bone window images in a 48-year-old female.MRI images of the same patient 1 year later show the lesion have grown and appear as T2 hyperintense lesion (c), T1 hypointense lesion (d, e) which shows heterogeneous enhancement after contrast administration (f).

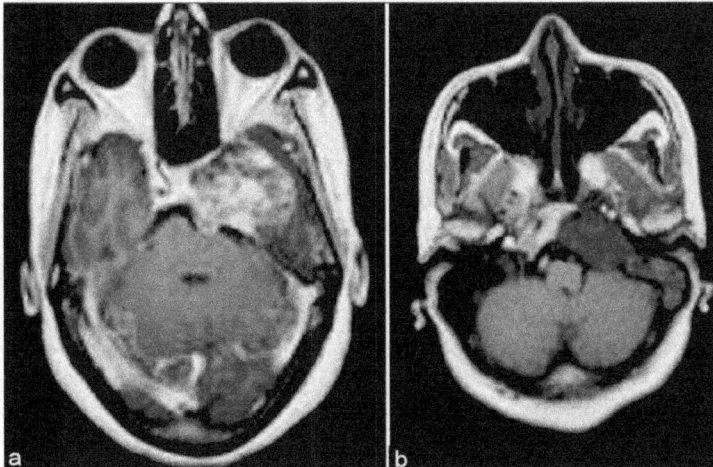

Figure 4.
Chondrosarcoma: (a) Postcontrast T_1-weighted axial image shows heterogeneous enrichment of lesion. (b) Figure showing T_1-weighted axial image: Lesion is hypointense on this image.

CT and MRI are essential to decide the tumor localization, as well as the degree of tumor development and the treatment logic, is to maximize tumor resection with reduced morbidity. On susceptibility-weighted imaging the chordoma show multiple areas of blooming which is a nonspecific finding and diffusion-weighted imaging can help to differentiate the conventional vs. dedifferentiated based on cut-off values of apparent diffusion coefficient.

6.2 Histopathology

The histopathological type of chordoma (i.e., classic (conventional), chondroid, and dedifferentiated) predicts the prognosis of this tumor. Chondroid chordoma appears in locales where the stroma takes after hyaline cartilage and neoplastic, occasionally physaliphorous cells develop in lacunae. The chondroid variant of chordoma and myxoid chondrosarcoma of cranium base are uncommon tumors and possess the same anatomic location, the clinical presentation sometimes coming about in their amalgamation [19]. But Chordoma and chondrosarcoma have particular histologic and immunohistologic highlights that generally permit for their precise refinement.

Cranium base chordomas emerge from remnants of the primitive notochord at the spheno-occipital synchondrosis, though chondrosarcoma begin from primitive mesenchymal cells or from the embryonic rest of the cartilaginous matrix of the skull. Using immune-histochemical staining they can be differentiated and pathological aspects can be studied. Chondrosarcoma is encompassed of cartilage with pleomorphic chondrocytes [24]. Chordomas comprise uniform cells containing small-oval, eccentric nuclei with prominent chromatin and physaliferous cells which can be identified in histopathology. Chondroid chordoma also possesses a cartilaginous component.

Histologically, chondrosarcomas are considered by a profuse hyaline sort of cartilaginous stroma and the presence of a neoplastic chondrocyte populace. Chondrocytes have an unnoticeable cytoplasm and a small, dark nucleus with fine chromatin. Invasion of the hard trabeculae could be a histological highlight of malignancy. It is strongly identified that chondrosarcomas illustrate recognizable histological grades of separation. Based on mitotic activity, cellularity, atypia, and size of the nucleus, World Health Organization (WHO) presented it in 3 groups namely grade I (well-differentiated), grade II (moderately differentiated), and grade III (poorly differentiated) [25]. Chondrosarcoma grade I and grade II show a better outcome while chondrosarcoma grade III is related with a high recurrence rate as well as metastases. Myxoid chondrosarcoma may be an uncommon mesenchymal soft-tissue malignancy of putative chondrocytic differentiation. Intermittent plain cartilage formation, positivity for S-100 protein, and ultrastructural examination have bolstered this view. In any case, most extraskeletal myxoid chondrosarcomas (EMCs) don't appear chondroid tissue arrangement, and S-100 protein is found in much less common than has been detailed. For the most part, utilizing matrix proteins as markers of mesenchymal cell differentiation explored the biochemical matrix composition and cellular phenotype of the tumor cells in illustrative specimens [26]. Extraskeletal myxoid chondrosarcoma comprises most likely primitive mesenchymal cells with focal, multidirectional differentiation. Chondrocytic differentiation is an abnormal aspect within the range of differentiation patterns displayed by these lesions.

EMC may be a very rare sarcoma subtype that usually ascends in the extremities, in spite of the fact that it can begin from any anatomic location and there are reports of primary EMC of the bone. EMC may occur anywhere exterior to the hard skeleton, synovial layer and the neurocranium and once in a while inside the bones. The histopathologic range of EMC ranges from lesions with densely packed rounded cells to those composed of cords of cells.

Chordomas show up as thick, multi-lobulated, semi-translucent greyish tumors and usually, lesions are 2–5 cm in measure [27]. In typical chordomas, the cells incline to be orchestrated in a set with a pale matrix of mucopolysaccharide with a specific physaliphorous appearance and in development, typical chordomas contain necrosis zone, hemorrhage, and bone trabeculae. Sometimes chondroid chordomas may look like low-grade chondrosarcomas and with the assistance of immune-histochemical observation, these tumors can be distinguished from others [8].

In chondroid chordoma combination of both chordoid and chondroid cells are found. Just in the case of chondromas, some free lying monomorphic cells having blurry cell borders along with faintly stained cell nuclei are usually observed lying within lacunary structures in a background of myxoid material. On histology, chondroid chordomas appear with physaliphorous cells admixed with epithelial cells (characteristic morphology of chordomas) in addition to cartilaginous background. High mitotic activity is also found in the case of chondrosarcomas. Chondromas are uncommon within the pelvis region and ordinarily hypocellular, however, it can be cellular and cytologically atypical. With the assistance of immunohistochemistry, we can differentiate these types of cancer. Prognosis depends on the degree of spread, the treatment choice chosen. Progress in the field of molecular genetics and epigenetics of chordoma and chondrosarcoma, have essentially refined the molecular concept of oncogenesis and hope in coming days it will advance in diagnosis and therapy.

6.3 Differential diagnosis

Chordoma and chondroid chordoma both are immune positive for epithelial markers cytokeratin (CK) and epithelial membrane antigen (EMA), though chondrosarcoma is negative for both [28]. Chordoma show up comparable to fetal notochord on both light and electron microscopy and are immune-histochemically and ultrastructurally similar. Chordoma of the cranium base starts at the spheno-occipital intersection and in soft tissues, they may be encapsulated in contrast to the bony lesion. In microscopy it appears as pseudo-encapsulated by fibrous strands making dense hylanized septa or thin septa creating lobules. Lobules show up as an area of vacuolated physaliferous cells and the sheets of cells contain intracytoplasmic mucin (**Figure 5**). In chondrosarcomas, immunehistochemical stains are negative for CK and EMA and positive for S-100 protein and Vimentin [15].

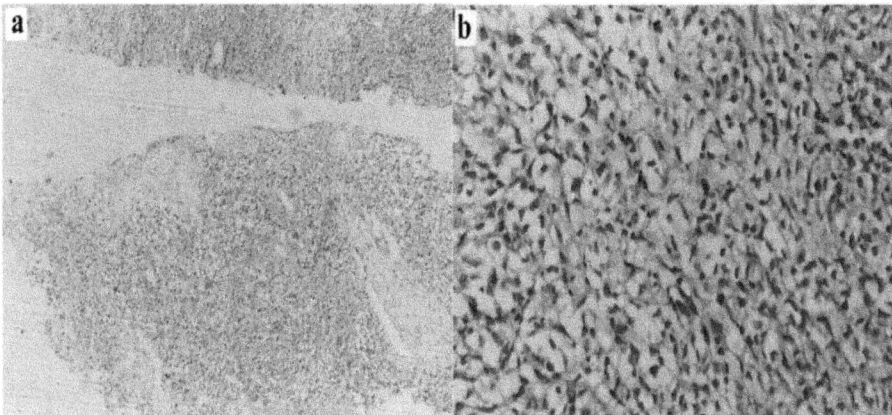

Figure 5.
Photomicrographs from a case of chordoma a) Tumor cells with the lobular arrangement are separated by fibrous septae (microscopic field with 100X in hematoxylin and eosin stain) b) Large bubbly-looking tumor cells with stellate-shaped nucleus and presence of physaliphorous-like cells (microscopic field with 200X in hematoxylin and eosin stain).

All chondroid and nonchondroid chordomas are positive for cytokeratin and vimentin and in most of the cases they are positive for S-100, EMA, neuron specifi-cenolase (NSE), and carcinoembryonic antigen (CEA). Neoplastic cells within the chondroid zones are stained similarly to those within the tumors. All chondrosar-comas are negative for cytokeratin, EMA, and CEA and are positive for vimentin and S-100. Chowhan et al., 2012 detailed the histological features of chondrosar-comas as a lobular lesional component including large cells with round to mildly pleomorphic vesicular nuclei along with abundant vacuolated cytoplasm lying on a mucomyxoid background (**Figure 6**) [4]. The immune-histochemical positivity of the tumor component for the S100 protein and Vimentin (**Figure 7**) and negative for EMA and CK favored the diagnosis of the myxoid variant of chondrosarcoma over chondroid chordoma [4].

IHC marker Brachyury may is used which is a very precise diagnostic marker for chordomas [29]. Other tumors don't show expression of this protein; hence it can be used as a diagnostic marker for chordomas [30]. It was also found that some differentiated zones of chordomas may show a loss of brachyury immune-reactivity [31]. Synaptophysin and Desmin can be used for staining purposes which is less

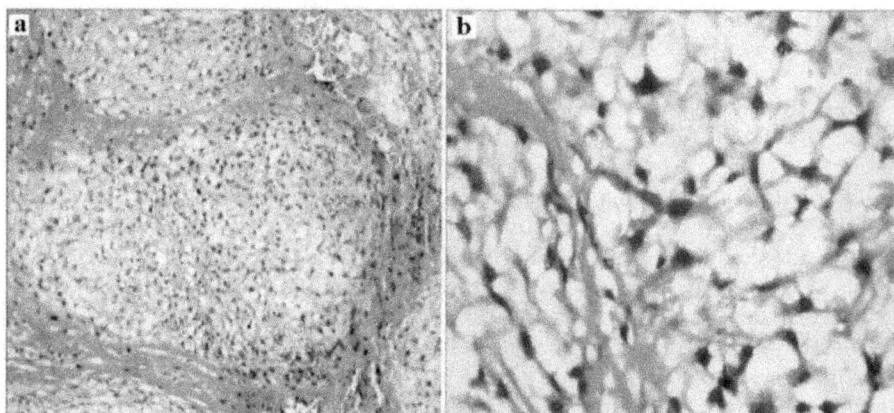

Figure 6.
Photomicrographs from a case of a myxoid variant of Chondrosarcoma) Tumor cells with the lobular arrangement are separated by fibrous septae (microscopic field with 200X in hematoxylin and eosin stain) b) Large bubbly-looking tumor cells with stellate-shaped nucleus and presence of physaliphorous-like cells (microscopic field with 400X in hematoxylin and eosin stain).

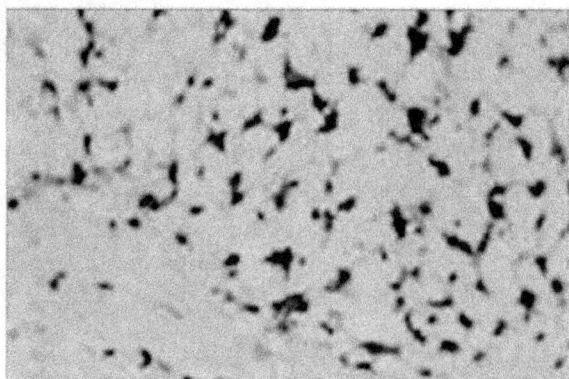

Figure 7.
Myxoid variant of chondrosarcoma showing cytoplasmic positivity for vimentin (microscopic field with 400X).

pathologically explored. Focal glial fibrillary acid protein (GFAP) immune-reactivity study is another technique that can be explored. Oliveira and his colleagues studied extraskeletal myxoid chondrosarcoma cells with immune reactivity reaction for smooth muscle actin, cytokeratin, polyclonal carcinoembryonic antigen (pCEA), and MIC2 [15]. They have found that all experimental tumor samples lacked the immunoreactivity of the said compounds.

For the histological study of collagen, Masson–Goldner staining may be used [26] as we know collagen is a very important component to study chondroid tumors [26]. Researchers have used to find suitable immune histochemical markers for assisting in the differential diagnosis between chordoma and other tumors with chordoid morphology with biomarkers like GFAP, D2–40, pan-cytokeratin (panCK) etc. Chordoma typically shows positive for panCK and negative for GFAP and D2–40; while chondrosarcoma reveals positive for D2–40, and negative for panCK, and GFAP [32]. To assess the proliferative activity of tumors, Ki-67 immunohistochemistry can be done [33].

7. Management

The primary modality of treatment of chordoma is maximal safe surgical excision of the tumor. This is to ensure maximal cytoreduction & minimizing the morbidity. In most larger-sized tumors complete excision is not technically possible, so some form of adjuvant radiotherapy (preferably with Proton Beam Therapy) is needed [34]. The indications for molecular targeted therapy in chordoma patients are to a great extent based on a number of imminent clinical trials, retrospective studies, and case reports [35]. In any case, the suitability and safety of molecularly targeted therapy regimens in chordoma patients and the fundamental molecular mechanisms, need more efficient research and clinical investigation. Subsequently, novel therapeutic strategies are required to drag out patients' survival and make strides in the quality of lifespan. Pathologically, chordoma emerges from remaining notochord cells inside the vertebral frame, as confirmed on the premise of molecular and immuno-genetic biomarkers [36].

In view of their un-accessible location in the clivus and their cell of origin from the remnants of notochord the Endonasal-Endoscopic surgical Approach (EEA) to these lesions offers an optimal cure [37, 38]. This approach gives the surgeon the most direct access to these tumors in contrast to the open transcranial/facial microscopic approaches which has more morbidity. However, the endoscopic approach requires a higher skill with a steep learning curve for the surgeons. Moreover, as these tumors are locally aggressive, in case of incomplete resection of these tumors, recurrence is the rule [39]. In certain cases, the tumors are large invading the dura mater and very often cause encasement of major intracranial arteries like internal carotid and basilar arteries, etc. In such cases, it is prudent to leave a sleeve of tumor around these critical structures to reduce postoperative morbidity. In this situation other modalities of treatment like proton beam external irradiation offer better locoregional control of the disease [40]. The advantages of proton beam radiotherapy is a very short dose fall-out effect of the proton beams, which helps a better disease control with limited side-effects on the critical structure like the brainstem. However, the proton beam external radiation is very expensive and not available in many centers [41].

7.1 Targeted therapy

Molecular targeted therapy (**Figure 8**) in chordoma incorporates a) erlotinib, lapatinib, gefitinib, and cetuximab against epidermal growth factor receptor (EGFR) and erbB-2/human epidermal growth factor receptor 2 (HER2/neu); b)

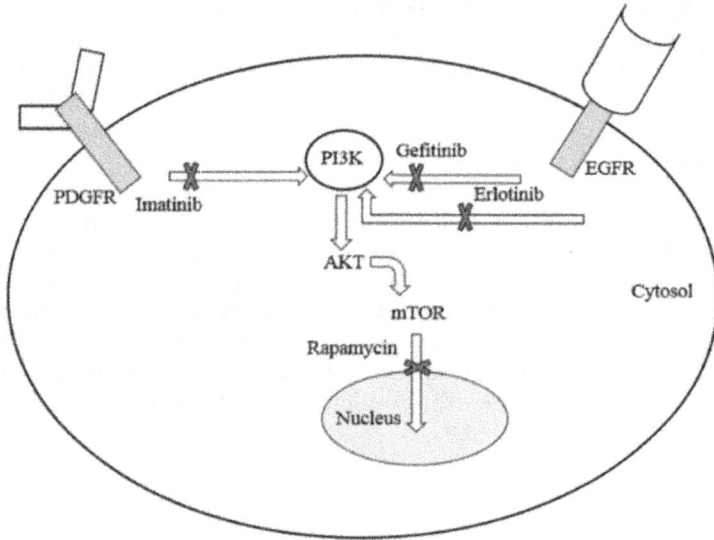

Figure 8.
Molecular targeted therapy in Chordoma using some inhibitor of the major signaling pathway that triggers for the progression of Chordoma [42].

imatinib and dasatinib against platelet-derived growth factor receptors (PDGFR) and stem cell factor receptor [43]; c) sorafenib, pazopanib, and sunitinib that target angiogenic components like vascular endothelial growth factor receptor [44]; and d) temsirolimus and sirolimus that target the phosphoinositide 3- kinase (PI3K)/ AKT/mammalian target of rapamycin (mTOR) pathway [42].

The hairy/enhancer-of-split related with YRPW motif 1 (HEY1; on 8q21.13) gene and the nuclear receptor coactivator 2 (NCOA2; on 8q13.3) [HEY1- NCOA2] gene combination has been recognized in mesenchymal chondrosarcoma [45]. Extraskeletal myxoid chondrosarcoma is additionally a slow-growing soft-tissue tumor containing conspicuous myxoid degeneration and described by extended clinical course despite higher rates of local recurrence as well as metastases. It is characterized by t(9;22)(q22;q12), combining Ewing sarcoma breakpoint region 1 (EWSR1). Other translocation accomplices to Nuclear Receptor Subfamily 4 Group A Member 3 (NR4A3) incorporate TATA-Box Binding Protein Associated Factor 15 (TAF15) and Transcription Factor 12 (TCF12) [46].

Chordomas are rare tumors that are notoriously refractory to chemotherapy and radiotherapy and the problems of handling aggressive and refractory chordoma have motivated the study of the biological foundations of this disease [11]. Molecular targeted therapy is an alternative way for the treatment of advanced chordoma [11]. The choice of molecular targeted inhibitors for patients with advanced or relapsed chordoma ought to be based on gene mutation screening and immunohistochemistry. Monotherapy with molecularly targeted inhibitors is suggested as the first-line of administration, and combination treatment may be the choice for drug-resistant chordoma. The brachyury vaccine may be a promising strategy and have a great prospect.

7.2 Radiotherapy

Patients with resectable chordomas, usually radiation therapy [RT] (preoperative, postoperative, or intraoperative) are utilized in conjunction with surgery to improve local control and disease-free survival. For treating spinal/sacral and clival/skull base chordomas, various retrospective studies and case series have demonstrated enhanced local control and disease-free survival with combined surgical/RT treatments [47, 48]. A meta-analysis of 464 individuals with cranial chordoma found a 68 percent recurrence rate and average/median disease-free survival of 23 and 45 months, respectively, in a meta-analysis [49]. In the treatment of patients with low-grade skull-based and cervical spine chondrosarcoma, proton beam RT, alone or in combination with photon beam RT, has been linked to excellent local tumor reduction and long-term survival. Carbon ion RT has also been shown to have a high local control rate in patients with chondrosarcoma of the skull [50], as well as other unresectable chondrosarcomas [51].

In both cranial and extracranial chordomas, specialized methods such as intensity-modulated radiation therapy (IMRT) and stereotactic radiosurgery (SRS)/stereotactic radiotherapy (SRT) have been linked to good local control rates [52]. Computed tomography (CT) is used to detect bone deterioration and calcifications in skull base chordomas, whereas magnetic resonance imaging (MRI) is used to define the tumor margin from the brain, characterize the position and extension of the tumor into the neighboring soft tissue structure, and visualize blood vessels [53]. When compared to CT, MRI gives a more precise and superior contrast with surrounding soft tissue, making it useful for assessing recurrent or metastatic lesions [54].

8. Prognosis

Weber and his colleagues have recognized histology, gross tumor volume, and brain compression as prognostic feature for local control for chondrosarcomas and chordomas as well as overall survival (OS) based on multivariate investigation [55]. Dedifferentiated chordomas usually display a poor prognosis and this subtype contains a 60% 3-year OS compared to an 89.4% 3-year OS for classical chordomas [8]. Bloch and his colleagues have revealed that grade III chondrosarcomas appear with aggressive behavior and are related with the most reduced survival rates [56]. They calculated a 5-year mortality rate was 11.5% in a systematic review of 560 patients with intracranial chondrosarcomas and median survival time of 2 years. The conventional and chondroid variants of chordoma have a favorable long-term prognosis, with a 3-year survival rate of 90% [57]. The dedifferentiated subtype shows aggressive behavior and the 3-year overall survival rate is around 60% [58].

9. Future aspects

Chordoma may be a malignant tumor with a few confusing highlights, such as its origin, and its neighborhood invasiveness, and moderate aggressive character. To conclude, in spite of the fact that the myxoid variation of chondrosarcoma and chondroid chordoma are comparative in a few viewpoints, they vary in their origin. Cranium base myxoid chondrosarcoma carries an extraordinarily more favorable result with negligible recurrence though chordomas counting its chondroid variant illustrates an aggressive clinical course with consistently destitute outcome after disease recurrence. Radiotherapy is usually suggested after surgery in chordoma, while resection of the tumor suffices in the myxoid variant of chondrosarcoma. Immunohistochemistry is the most common application of immunostaining and it is also widely used to differentiate chondrosarcoma and chordoma and understand the scattering and localization of biomarkers and differentially expressed proteins in different cellular parts of chondrosarcoma and chordoma.

In spite of the advance in current surgical strategies and some encouraging results with the use of targeted therapy, control of the disease and long-term patient prognosis are still not satisfactory. However, understanding of the molecular basis of chordoma pathophysiology hopefully will give us a better understanding to improve the prognosis of this rare malignancy. Currently, surgical resection is the favored treatment for chordoma, whereas recent advances are focused on curative treatment and advanced radiotherapy may play for the treatment of chordoma, and surgery will be done only for the most advanced cases of chordoma.

Acknowledgements

The author acknowledges the contribution of Dr. Rabi Narayan Sahu, Professor, Neurosurgery, AIIMS, Bhubaneswar for his inputs regarding management protocol, Dr. Rakesh Kumar Gupta, Assistant Professor, Pathology & Laboratory Medicine, AIIMS, Raipur for the contribution of histopathology photomicrograph and Dr. Suman Kumar Ray, PhD (Molecular Biology) for help in writing the manuscript.

Conflict of interest

The authors declare no conflict of interest.

Abbreviations

CK	Cytokeratin
CT	Computed tomography
EGF	Epidermal growth factor
PD-1	Programmed cell death protein 1
PI3K	Phosphoinositide 3-kinase
SWI/SNF	Switch/Sucrose non-fermentable gene
CDK4/6	Cyclin-dependent kinases 4 and 6
CDKN2A	Cyclin-dependent kinase inhibitor 2A
CEA	Carcinoembryonic antigen
COL2A1	Collagen Type II Alpha 1 Chain
EGFR	Epidermal growth factor receptor
EMA	Epithelial membrane antigen
EMC	Extraskeletal myxoid chondrosarcomas
EWSR1	Ewing sarcoma breakpoint region 1
Gal9	Galectin-9
GFAP	Glial fibrillary acid protein
HER2	Human epidermal growth factor receptor 2
HEY1	Hairy/enhancer-of-split related with YRPW motif 1
HIF-1α	Hypoxia-inducible factor-1α
IGF-1	Insulin-like growth factor 1
IHC	Immunohistochemistry
IMRT	Intensity-modulated radiation therapy
MCS	Mesenchymal chondrosarcoma
miRNAs	MicroRNA
MRI	Magnetic resonance imaging
mTOR	Mammalian target of rapamycin

NCOA2	Nuclear receptor coactivator 2
NR4A3	Nuclear Receptor Subfamily 4 Group A Member 3
NSE	Neuron specific enolase
OS	Overall survival
panCK	Pan-cytokeratin
pCEA	Polyclonal carcinoembryonic antigen
PDGF	Platelet-derived growth factor
PDGFR	Platelet-derived growth factor receptors
PD-L1	Programmed cell death ligand 1
PIK3CA	Phosphatidylinositol-4,5-Bisphosphate 3-Kinase catalytic subunit Alpha
PTEN	Phosphate and tensin homolog
RTK	Receptor tyrosine kinases
RUNX2	Runt-related transcription factor 2
SRS	Stereotactic radiosurgery
SRT	Stereotactic radiotherapy
TAF15	TATA Box Binding Protein Associated Factor 15
TBXT	T-box transcription factor T
TIL	Tumor-infiltrating lymphocytes
TIM3	T-cell immunoglobulin and mucin-domain 3
VEGF	Vascular endothelial growth factor
WHO	World Health Organization

Author details

Amit Kumar Chowhan[1*] and Pavan Kumar G. Kale[2]

1 Department of Pathology and Lab Medicine, All India Institute of Medical Sciences, Raipur, Chhattisgarh, India

2 Radiology, Sri Venkateswara Institute of Medical Sciences, Tirupati, Andhra Pradesh, India

*Address all correspondence to: chowhanpath@aiimsraipur.edu.in

IntechOpen

References

[1] Topsakal C, Bulut S, Erol FS, Ozercan I, Yildirim H. Chordoma of the thoracic spine. Case report. Neurologia Medico-Chirurgica (Tokyo). 2002;**42**: 175-180

[2] Chigurupati P, Venkatesan V, Thiyagarajan M, Vikram A, Kiran K. Sacrococcygeal chordoma presenting as a retro rectal tumour. International Journal of Surgery Case Reports. 2014;**5**:714-716

[3] Erazo IS, Galvis CF, Aguirre LE, Iglesias R, Abarca LC. Clival chondroid chordoma: A case report and review of the literature. Cureus. 2018;**10**:3381

[4] Chowhan AK, Rukmangadha N, Patnayak R, Bodapati CM, Bodagala VL, Reddy MK. Myxoid chondrosarcoma of sphenoid bone. Journal of Neurosciences in Rural Practice. 2012;**3**:395-398

[5] Virchow RL. Untersuchungen über die Entwickelung des Schädelgrundes-imgesunden und krankhaftenZustande: und über den Einflussderselben auf Schädelform, Gesichtsbildung und Gehirnbau. Berlin: G Reimer; 1857

[6] Hirsch EF, Ingals M. Sacrococcygeal-chordoma. Journal of the American Medical Association. 1923;**80**:1369-1370

[7] Williams LW. The later development of the notochord in mammals. The American Journal of Anatomy. 1908;**8**: 251-284

[8] Kremenevski N, Schlaffer SM, Coras R, Kinfe TM, Graillon T, Buchfelder M. Skull base chordomas and chondrosarcomas. Neuroendocrinology. 2020;**110**:836-847

[9] Sun X, Hornicek F, Schwab JH. Chordoma: An update on the pathophysiology and molecular mechanisms. Current Reviews in Musculoskeletal Medicine. 2015;**8**: 344-352

[10] Yamaguchi T, Suzuki S, Ishiiwa H, Shimizu K, Ueda Y. Benign notochordal cell tumors: A comparative histological study of benign notochordal cell tumors, classic chordomas, and notochordal vestiges of fetal inter-vertebral discs. The American Journal of Surgical Pathology. 2004; **28**(6):756-761

[11] Hoffman SE, Al Abdulmohsen SA, Gupta S, Hauser BM, Meredith DM, Dunn IF, et al. Translational windows in chordoma: A target appraisal. Frontiers in Neurology. 2020;**11**:657

[12] Bai J, Shi J, Li C, Wang S, Zhang T, Hua X, et al. Whole genome sequencing of skull-Base chordoma reveals genomic alterations associated with recurrence and chordoma-specific survival. Nature Communications. 2021;**12**:757

[13] Chow WA. Chondrosarcoma: Biology, genetics, and epigenetics. F1000Research. 2018;7:1-9

[14] Meng T, Jin J, Jiang C, Huang R, Yin H, Song D, et al. Molecular targeted therapy in the treatment of chordoma: A systematic review. Frontiers in Oncology. 2019;**9**:30

[15] Oliveira A, Sebo T, McGrory J, Gaffey TA, Rock MG, Nascimento AG, et al. Extraskeletal myxoid chondrosarcoma: A clinicopathologic, immunohistochemical, and ploidy analysis of 23 cases. Modern Pathology. 2000;**13**:900-908

[16] Roberti F, Sekhar LN, Jones RV, Wright DC. Intradural cranial chordoma: A rare presentation of an uncommon tumor. Surgical experience and review of the literature. Journal of Neurosurgery. 2007;**106**:270-274

[17] Asioli S, Zoli M, Guaraldi F, Sollini G, Bacci A, Gibertoni D, et al. Peculiar pathological, radiological and

clinical features of skull-base de-differentiated chordomas. Results from a referral centre case-series and literature review. Histopathology. 2020;**76**:731-739

[18] Singh AK, Srivastava AK, Sardhara J, Bhaisora KS, Das KK, Mehrotra A, et al. Skull base bony lesions: Management nuances; a retrospective analysis from a Tertiary Care Centre. Asian Journal of Neurosurgery. 2017;**12**:506-513

[19] Almefty K, Pravdenkova S, Colli BO, Al-Mefty O, Gokden M. Chordoma and chondrosarcoma: Similar, but quite different, skull base tumors. Cancer. 2007;**110**:2457-2467

[20] Erdem E, Angtuaco EC, Van Hemert R, Park JS, Al-Mefty O. Comprehensive review of intracranial chordoma. Radiographics. 2003;**23**: 995-1009

[21] Chordoma MM. Antibodies to epithelial membrane antigen and carcinoembryonic antigen in differential diagnosis. Archives of Pathology & Laboratory Medicine. 1984;**108**:891-892

[22] Persson S, Kindblom LG, Angervall L. Classical and chondroidchordoma. A light-microscopic, histochemical, ultrastructural and immunohisto-chemical analysis of the various cell types. Pathology, Research and Practice. 1991;**187**:828-828

[23] Soule E, Baig S, Fiester P, Holtzman A, Rutenberg M, Tavanaiepour D, et al. Current management and image review of skull base chordoma: What the radiologist needs to know. Journal of Clinical Imaging Science. 2021;**11**:46

[24] Boehme KA, Schleicher SB, Traub F, Rolauffs B. Chondrosarcoma: A rare misfortune in aging human cartilage? The role of stem and progenitor cells in proliferation, malignant degeneration and

therapeutic resistance. International Journal of Molecular Sciences. 2018;**19**: 311

[25] Hogendoorn PCW, Bovée JV, Nielsen GP. Chondrosarcoma (grades I-III), including primary and secondary variants and periosteal chondrosarcoma. In: Fletcher CD, Bridge JA, Hogendoorn PC, et al., editors. World Health Organization Classification of Tumours. Pathology and Genetics of Tumours of Soft Tissue and Bone. 4th ed. Lyon: IARC Press; 2013. pp. 264-268

[26] Aigner T, Oliveira AM, Nascimento AG. Extra skeletal myxoid chondrosarcomas do not show a chondrocytic phenotype. Modern Pathology. 2004;**17**:214-221

[27] Weber AL, Liebsch NJ, Sanchez R. Chordoma of the skull base. Neuroimaging Clinics of North America. 1994;**4**:515-527

[28] Metcalfe C, Muzaffar J, Kulendra K, Sanghera P, Shaw S, Shad A, et al. Chordomas and chondrosarcomas of the skull base: Treatment and outcome analysis in a consecutive case series of 24 patients. World Journal of Surgical Oncology. 2021;**19**:68

[29] Vujovic S, Henderson S, Presneau N, Odell E, Jacques TS, Tirabosco R, et al. Brachyury, a crucial regulator of notochordal development, is a novel biomarker for chordomas. The Journal of Pathology. 2006;**209**:157-165

[30] Barresi V, Ieni A, Branca G, Tuccari G. Brachyury: A diagnostic marker for the differential diagnosis of chordoma and hemangioblastoma versus neoplastic histological mimickers. Disease Markers. 2014;**2014**:514753

[31] Jambhekar NA, Rekhi B, Thorat K, Dikshit R, Agrawal M, Puri A. Revisiting chordoma with brachyury, a "new age" marker: Analysis of a validation study on 51 cases. Archives of Pathology & Laboratory Medicine. 2010;**134**:1181-1187

[32] Cho HY, Lee M, Takei H, Dancer J, Ro JY, Zhai QJ. Immunohistochemical comparison of chordoma with chondrosarcoma, myxopapillary-ependymoma, and chordoid meningioma. Applied Immunohisto-chemistry & Molecular Morphology. 2009;**17**:131-138

[33] Horbinski C, Oakley GJ, Cieply K, Mantha GS, Nikiforova MN, Dacic S, et al. The prognostic value of Ki-67, p53, epidermal growth factor receptor, 1p36, 9p21, 10q23, and 17p13 in skull base chordomas. Archives of Pathology & Laboratory Medicine. 2010;**134**:1170-1176

[34] Amichetti M, Cianchetti M, Amelio D, Enrici RM, Minniti G. Proton therapy in chordoma of the base of the skull: A systematic review. Neurosurgical Review. 2009;**32**:403-416

[35] Lebellec L, Chauffert B, Blay JY, Le Cesne A, Chevreau C, Bompas E, et al. Advanced chordoma treated by first-line molecular targeted therapies: Outcomes and prognostic factors. A retrospective study of the French Sarcoma Group (GSF/GETO) and the Association des Neuro-Oncologuesd'Expression Francaise (ANOCEF). European Journal of Cancer. 2017;**79**:119-128

[36] Tarpey PS, Behjati S, Young MD, Martincorena I, Alexandrov LB, Farndon SJ, et al. The driver landscape of sporadic chordoma. Nature Communications. 2017;**8**:890

[37] Fernandez–Miranda JC, Gardner PA, Snyderman CH, Devaney KO, Mendenhall WM, Suárez C, et al. Clival chordomas: A pathological, surgical, and radiotherapeutic review. Head & Neck. 2014;**36**:892-906

[38] Fraser JF, Nyquist GG, Moore N, Anand VK, Schwartz TH. Endoscopic endonasal transclival resection of chordomas: Operative technique, clinical outcome, and review of the literature. Journal of Neurosurgery. 2010;**112**: 1061-1069

[39] Koutourousiou M, Gardner PA, Tormenti MJ, Henry SL, Stefko ST, Kassam AB, et al. Endoscopic endonasal approach for resection of cranial base chordomas: Outcomes and learning curve. Neurosurgery. 2012;**71**(3):614-625

[40] Jahangiri A, Chin AT, Wagner JR, Kunwar S, Ames C, Chou D, et al. Factors predicting recurrence after resection of Clival chordoma using variable surgical approaches and radiation modalities. Neurosurgery. 2015;**76**(2):179-186

[41] Peeters A, Grutters JP, Pijls-Johannesma M, Reimoser S, De Ruysscher D, Severens JL, et al. How costly is particle therapy? Cost analysis of external beam radiotherapy with carbon-ions, protons and photons. Radiotherapy and Oncology. 2010;**95**(1):45-53

[42] Di Maio S, Yip S, Al Zhrani GA, Alotaibi F, Al Turki A, Kong E, et al. Novel targeted therapies in chordoma: An update. Therapeutics and Clinical Risk Management. 2015;**11**:873-883

[43] Stacchiotti S, Tamborini E, Lo Vullo S, Bozzi F, Messina A, Morosi C, et al. Phase II study on lapatinib in advanced EGFR-positive chordoma. Annals of Oncology. 2013;**24**:1931-1936

[44] Jagersberg M, El Rahal A, Dammann P, Merkler D, Weber DC, Schaller K. Clival chordoma: A single-centre outcome analysis. Acta Neurochirurgica (Wein). 2017;**159**: 1815-1823

[45] Wang L, Motoi T, Khanin R, Olshen A, Mertens F, Bridge J, et al. Identification of a novel, recurrent HEY1- NCOA2 fusion in mesenchymal-chondrosarcoma based on a genome-wide screen of exon-level expression data. Genes, Chromosomes & Cancer. 2012;**51**(2):127-139

[46] Hisaoka M, Ishida T, Imamura T, Hashimoto H. TFG is a novel fusion

partner of NOR1 in Extraskeletal myxoid chondrosarcoma. Genes, Chromosomes & Cancer. 2004;**40**:325-328

[47] Indelicato DJ, Rotondo RL, Begosh-Mayne D, Scarborough MT, Gibbs CP, Morris CG, et al. A prospective outcomes study of proton therapy for chordomas and chondrosarcomas of the spine. International Journal of Radiation Oncology, Biology, Physics. 2016;**95**: 297-303

[48] McDonald MW, Linton OR, Moore MG, Ting JY, Cohen-Gadol AA, Shah MV. Influence of residual tumor volume and radiation dose coverage in outcomes for clival chordoma. International Journal of Radiation Oncology, Biology, Physics. 2016;**95**:304-311

[49] Jian BJ, Bloch OG, Yang I, Han SJ, Aranda D, Tihan T, et al. Adjuvant radiation therapy and chondroidchordoma subtype are associated with a lower tumor recurrence rate of cranial chordoma. Journal of Neuro-Oncology. 2010;**98**:101-108

[50] Schulz-Ertner D, Nikoghosyan A, Hof H, Didinger B, Combs SE, Jäkel O, et al. Carbon ion radiotherapy of skull base chondrosarcomas. International Journal of Radiation Oncology, Biology, Physics. 2007;**67**: 171-177

[51] Imai R, Kamada T, Araki N; Working Group For Bone And Soft-Tissue Sarcomas. Clinical efficacy of carbon ion radiotherapy for unresectable chondrosarcomas. Anticancer Research. 2017;**37**:6959-6964

[52] Bugoci DM, Girvigian MR, Chen JC, Miller MM, Rahimian J. Photon-based fractionated stereotactic radiotherapy for postoperative treatment of skull base chordomas. American Journal of Clinical Oncology. 2013;**36**:404-410

[53] Weber AL, Liebsch NJ, Sanchez R, Sweriduk ST Jr. Chordomas of the skull base. Radiologic and clinical evaluation. Neuroimaging Clinics of North America. 1994;**4**:515-527

[54] Plathow C, Weber MA, Debus J, Kauczor HU. Imaging of sacral chordoma: Comparison between MRI and CT. Radiologe. 2005;**45**:63-68

[55] Weber DC, Malyapa R, Albertini F, Bolsi A, Kliebsch U, Walser M, et al. Long term outcomes of patients with skull-base low-grade Chondrosarcoma and chordoma patients treated with pencil beam scanning proton therapy. Radiotherapy and Oncology. 2016;**120**:169-174

[56] Bloch OG, Jian BJ, Yang I, Han SJ, Aranda D, Ahn BJ, et al. A systematic review of intracranial chondrosarcoma and survival. Journal of Clinical Neuroscience. 2009;**16**:1547-1551

[57] Chugh R, Tawbi H, Lucas DR, Biermann JS, Schuetze SM, Baker LH. Chordoma: The nonsarcoma primary bone tumor. The Oncologist. 2007;**12**: 1344-1350

[58] Casali PG, Stacchiotti S, Sangalli C, Olmi P, Gronchi A. Chordoma. Current Opinion in Oncology. 2007;**19**:367-370

Section 7

Orbital Surgery

Chapter 8

Extended Orbital Exenteration: A Step-by-Step Approach

Arsheed Hussain Hakeem, Hassaan Javaid,
Novfa Iftikhar and Usaamah Javaid

Abstract

Extended orbital exenteration is a highly disfiguring operation which entails complete removal of the orbital contents including periorbita, eyelids and involved surrounding bony walls with variations tailored to the specific clinical circumstances. The aim of such an extensive surgery is to achieve local control of the life-threatening progressive neoplasms, when other treatment modalities fail to achieve disease control. Eyelids can be preserved in posterior orbital pathology, while it may not be possible in neoplasms arising from the anterior eye tissues. Depending on the clinical circumstances, if the neoplasm is invading the surrounding bony orbit, the involved bony and soft tissue structures are removed en bloc to achieve complete resection (R0 resection). Although the steps of the orbital exenteration are well defined, the same is not true for extended orbital exenteration. We demonstrate the details of extended orbital exenteration in different clinical scenarios for the malignancy of orbit and periorbital tissues invading surrounding orbital walls.

Keywords: extended orbital exenteration, orbital neoplasms, paranasal sinuses, skin malignant tumors, reconstruction, rehabilitation

1. Introduction

Any ocular or periocular tumor, if neglected, can invade the orbit and raise the probability of various forms of orbital exenteration. Approximately 2–4% of the periocular malignancies invade the orbit and are candidates for orbital exenteration or extended procedures [1–6]. Frezzoti et al. classified orbital exenterations into subtotal, total and radical (**Table 1**) [7]. The radical resections or extended orbital exenteration have been classified as Type V (removal of bony walls) and VI (removal of bony walls and adjacent structures) (**Table 1**) [7]. Exenteration or its variations are psychologically and anatomically disfiguring, hence reserved to treat potentially life-threatening malignancies unresponsive to other treatments. Extended orbital exenteration has wide variations to the basic technique and is tailored to the clinical circumstances. These variations depend on saving or sacrificing different tissues within or around the orbit. Clinical and radiological findings guide the surgeon to tailor make the resection needed to completely remove the tumor with negative margins along with the selected sections of the orbital bone. Extended orbital exenteration, although highly disfiguring surgery, offers the best chance of cure as it aims to achieve local control of extensive disease when other treatment modalities fail to halt the progression of the disease [8]. The

Stage	Type	Surgical technique
Subtotal exenteration	I	Eyelids and palpebral and bulbar conjunctiva sparing
	II	Eyelids and palpebral conjunctiva sparing
	III	Eyelid skin and deeper muscle layer sparing
Total exenteration	IV	Eyelid resection
Radical exenteration	V	Resection of orbital cavity bones
	VI	Extension of adjacent structures

Source: Adapted from Frezzotti et al. [7].

Table 1.
Categorization of orbital exenteration based upon surgical technique.

basic technique is somewhat similar to the orbital exenteration which removes all orbital contents including the periorbita along with part or complete eyelids. But variations are tailor made depending on the extent of the disease as assessed by the CT or MRI scan [9, 10]. Eyelids may be spared if the pathology present posteriorly not infiltrating them [11]. We describe different indications and step by step approach to different clinical presentations of orbital tumors.

2. Indications

Any tumor arising from the globe or periocular tissues with involvement of orbital apex, full thickness periorbita or periosteum, retro-orbital fat, extraocular muscles, conjunctiva and sclera form an indication for orbital exenteration (**Table 2**). Different Tumors which result in orbital invasion are depicted in **Table 3**.

2.1 Malignant tumors arising from eyelids and surrounding skin

Basal cell carcinoma is the most common malignant skin tumor accounting for 90% these cases; squamous cell carcinoma and sebaceous gland carcinoma each comprising approximately 4–6% of cases [1–6, 8–13]. The reported incidence of orbital invasion in basal cell carcinoma is 1.6–2.5% and risk factors include multiple recurrences, large size, aggressive histological subtype like infiltrative and morpheic patterns, perineural spread, canthal location particularly the medial canthus and age over 70. The incidence of orbital invasion is high in squamous cell 5.9% and much higher in sebaceous gland carcinoma 6–45% [14, 15].

2.2 Malignant conjunctival tumors

Advanced and invasive conjunctival melanoma and ocular surface squamous cell carcinoma require orbital exenteration. Approximately 15% of ocular surface squamous cell carcinoma invade orbit as reported McKelvie et al. [16]. The rare variants of ocular surface carcinoma like mucoepidermoid or spindle cell carcinomas and are better controlled orbital exenteration [11].

2.3 Orbital sarcomas

Orbital rhabdomyosarcoma is presently treated with combination of radiotherapy and chemotherapy. Orbital exenteration may be indicated either in poor

Indications of orbital exenteration and extended procedures		
Primary tumors of globe with	I	Orbital apex
Malignant tumors arising from eyelids and surrounding skin with.	II	Invasion through periorbita
Orbital sarcomas with.	III	Involvement of retro-orbital fat
Lacrimal gland tumors with.		
Tumors of the paranasal sinuses and nose with.	IV	Extension into the extraocular muscles
Lacrimal sac tumors		
	V	Invasion of the conjunctiva or sclera
	VI	Extension of adjacent structures

Table 2.
Indications for orbital exenterations.

Different pathologies involving the orbit and peri-orbital tissues		
Periocular cutaneous malignant tumors	Basal cell carcinoma	
	Squamous cell carcinoma	
	Sebaceous gland carcinoma	
Conjunctival tumors	Ocular surface squamous cell carcinoma	Mucoepidermoid variant
		Spindle cell variant
	Malignant melanoma	
Choroidal melanoma	Choroidal melanoma with extra-scleral extension	
Sarcomas	Rhabdomyosarcoma post chemoradiation residual/recurrent	
Lacrimal gland tumors	Squamous cell carcinoma Transitional cell carcinoma Adenocarcinoma Mucoepidermoid carcinoma Adenoid cystic carcinoma Poorly differentiated carcinoma	
Lacrimal sac tumors	Squamous cell carcinoma Transitional cell carcinoma Adenocarcinoma Mucoepidermoid carcinoma Adenoid cystic carcinoma Poorly differentiated carcinoma	
Nose and paranasal sinus tumors	Carcinomas	
	Squamous cell carcinoma Adenocarcinoma Olfactory neuroblastoma, Malignant melanoma Adenoid cystic carcinoma	
	Sarcomas	
	Chondrosarcoma Rhabdomyosarcoma Osteosarcoma	
Invasive fungal infections	Sino-orbital aspergillosis involving retrobulbar tissues and the orbital apex	
	Sino orbital Mucormycosis involving retroorbital tissue and the orbital apex	

Table 3.
Common pathologies of eye and orbit.

responders or recurrent sarcomas. Alveolar soft part sarcomas may need upfront orbital exenteration with adjuvant radiotherapy.

2.4 Lacrimal gland tumors

Advanced adenoid cystic carcinoma of the lacrimal gland especially stage III and IV is an indication for orbital exenteration. Adenoid cystic carcinoma of the lacrimal gland is known to invade bone as well as demonstrate perineural invasion.

2.5 Tumors of the paranasal sinuses and nose

Paranasal sinuses and nose tumors may also require exenteration in case they extend to the orbital apex, complete thickness invasion through periorbita into posterior orbital fat, extension into the extraocular muscles and invasion of the bulbar conjunctiva or sclera.

2.6 Lacrimal sac tumors

Invasive neoplasms arising lacrimal sac like squamous cell, adenoid cystic carcinoma with infiltration into the orbit is an indication for orbital exenteration.

2.7 Invasive fungal infection

Uncontrolled invasive fungal infection like invasive aspergillosis or Mucor mycosis may need orbital exenteration for control.

3. Surgical technique

We will describe step by step approach of various forms of orbital exenterations. The basic procedure is lid sparing total orbital exenteration and other forms are modifications of this procedure. All orbital contents are removed in entirety with preservation of the major part of the upper and lower lids. Once again we are stressing the fact that any form orbital exenteration is a radical procedure with high degree of disfigurement and therefore should be only considered when there is a valid indication as mentioned above.

4. Total orbital exenteration-lid preserving

Lid preserving orbital exenteration is an excellent surgical procedure as it takes care of the challenge of providing a good concave stable skin cover over which customized prosthesis can be glued. If it is not oncologically safe to preserve eyelids, they can be sacrificed and orbital cavity can be lined by temporalis fascia/muscle, fore head flap or split-thickness skin graft. Some surgeons do advocate spontaneous granulation method, however healing by granulation takes a long time and needs intensive post-operative care. Lid sparing technique avoid these sequels provided this method is technically feasible. This method, popularized by Coston and Small, is the modification of total exenteration technique which preserve major parts of both the eye lids [17]. A transverse blepharorrhaphy is done to cover the orbit thus ensuing good cosmesis and fast healing. This method also spares orbicularis muscle which provides an excellent vascular supply to the skin flap enhancing early healing.

5. Steps

Orbital exenteration should be performed under general anesthesia. Incision is marked on closed eyelids approximately 2 mm beyond the eyelash line including medial and lateral canthus (**Figure 1**). A sterile gauze piece is placed in the cul de sac in conjunctival tumors to avoid maceration. The eyelid can be divided into two lamellae, namely, the anterior and the posterior. The anterior lamella consists of the skin and orbicularis muscle, while the posterior lamella is formed by tarsus and conjunctiva. Three traction sutures with 4–0 silk are placed through the upper and lower tarsi to provide traction on the orbital contents (**Figure 2A** and **B**). Incision is then made with radiofrequency probe, 15 no blade or cutting diathermy along the skin markings (**Figure 3A** and **B**). Further dissection is done in pre-septal plane, which avoids injury to orbital septum, especially important in the cases where tumor is present in the anterior orbit. This technique spared orbicularis muscle which provides an excellent vascular supply to the skin flap. Dissection is further continued with bipolar cautery till the orbital rim is reached (**Figure 4A** and **B**). The periosteum along the arcus marginalis or orbital rim is incised 360^0 (**Figure 5A** and **B**). Periosteal elevator is used to dissect the periosteum off the orbital rim and continued all the way to the orbital apex (**Figure 6**). Medially, along the superior orbital rim, superior orbital notch is encountered. The supra orbital neurovascular bundle is identified and cauterized (**Figure 7A** and **B**). On the medial wall, subperiosteal dissection is done from the anterior to the posterior lacrimal crest remaining medial to the lacrimal sac. Meticulous dissection is required here to avoid fracture of the thin lamella papyracea. Mostly periosteum can be easily

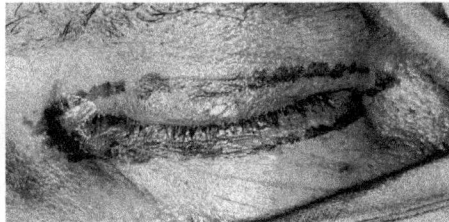

Figure 1.
The skin incision for the eyelid sparing orbital exenteration is made 2 mm behind the ciliary margin.

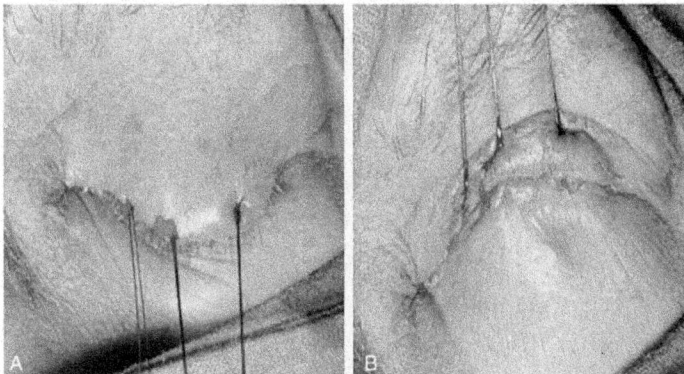

Figure 2.
Two or three traction sutures are placed through the upper and lower tarsi to provide traction on the orbital contents.

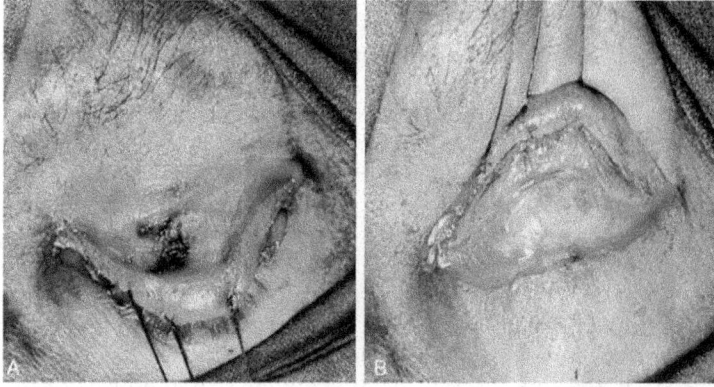

Figure 3.
Skin incision is made along the marked area using radiofrequency probe or 15 no blade or cutting diathermy.

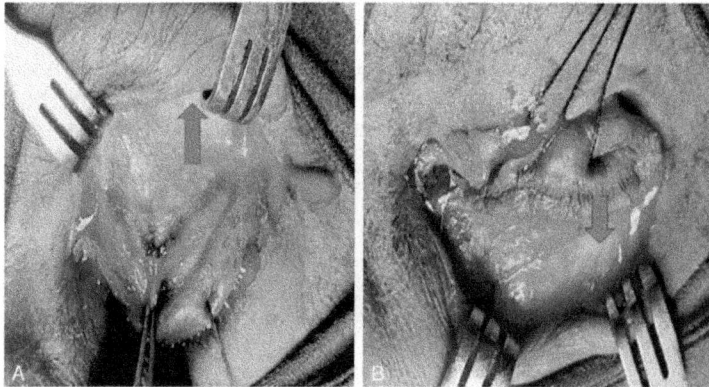

Figure 4.
Skin and orbicularis flaps are raised up to bony rim for 360°.

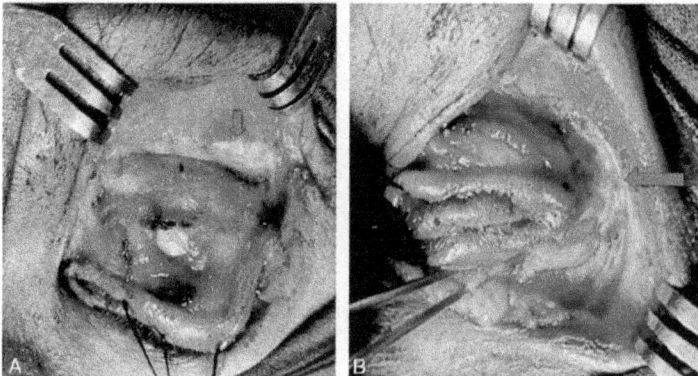

Figure 5.
The periosteum is incised for 360 degrees along the orbital margin.

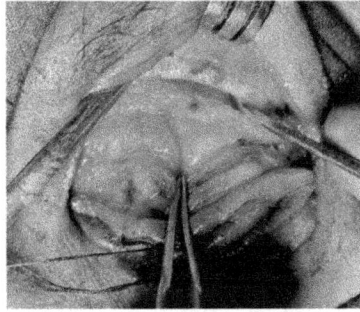

Figure 6.
The periosteum is elevated from orbital rim up to the apex of the orbit 360°.

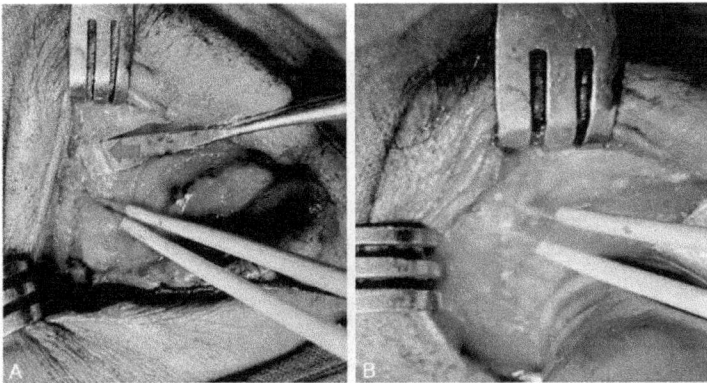

Figure 7.
Supra-orbital neurovascular bundle (arrow) is identified and cauterized.

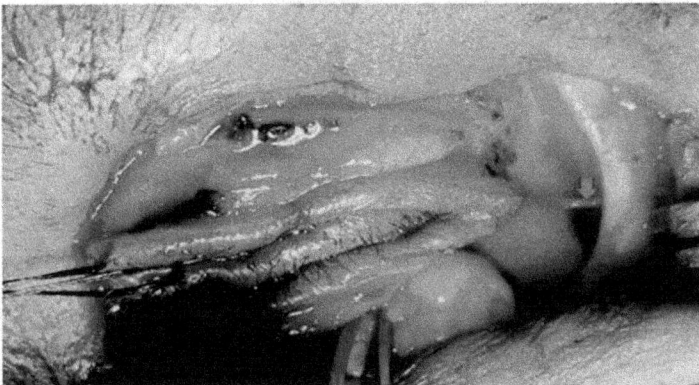

Figure 8.
Zygomatico- facial neurovascular bundle identified.

elevated as it is loosely adherent to orbital bones, except in certain locations like sutures and fissures where tight adhesions are encountered. Gentle dissection is carried out at these tight adhesions to avoid tearing of periosteum. Laterally, the frontozygomatic suture is identified and periosteum elevated to identify and zygomatico-facial and zygomatico- temporal neurovascular bundles which are then cauterized (**Figure 8**).

Floor of the orbit is thin and fragile like medial lamina papyracea and dissection has to be gentle so as not to fracture it or create a communication with maxillary sinus. As the lacrimal sac is approached by dissecting medial to it, nasolacrimal duct is divided with diathermy. The exposed end of the nasolacrimal duct is further cauterized with diathermy to obliterate it. This step decreases the risk by of post-operative fistula formation. Next, inferior orbital fissure is encountered and penetrating vessels are divided by cautery. After separation of the periosteum 360^0 from the from arcus marginalis to the orbital apex, a pair of curved enucleation scissors are introduced into the posterior orbit. With left hand traction is applied and with the right hand the optic nerve, the superior orbital contents and posterior orbital tissues are divided. Hemostasis is achieved by ice cold wet gauze, pressure and cautery. If necessary additional hemostasis is achieved by surgicel and bone wax. The empty socket is examined meticulously for any residual tumor tissue (**Figure 9**). Additional apical tissue can be resected if needed and complete

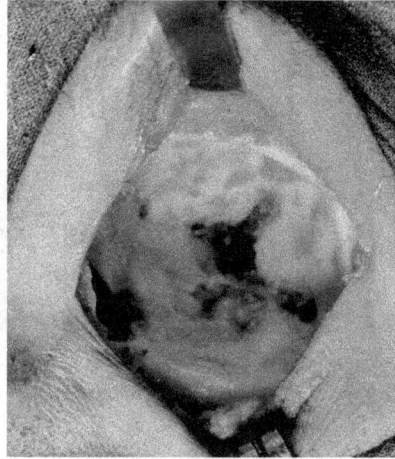

Figure 9.
View of the orbit after resection is complete.

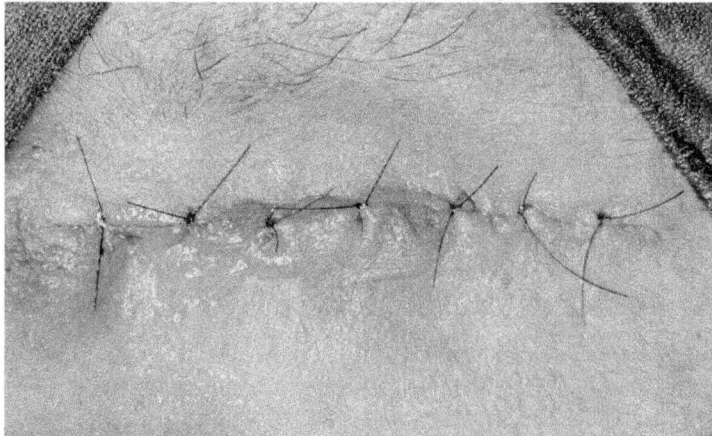

Figure 10.
Closure of the skin flaps of the orbit.

hemostasis achieved. Frozen section analysis can be done to assess adequacy of resection. The eyelid flaps are reapproximated with 4–0 vicryl for orbicularis and 6–0 ethilon for skin (**Figure 10**). Aspiration of the socket for blood or serum is done as and when required. Usually socket heals by 6 weeks and is ready for prosthesis placement by 8 weeks. The main advantage of the lid sparing is early wound healing, better cosmesis, and minimum patient morbidity.

6. Extended orbital exenteration

Extended orbital exenteration is a challenge to the surgeon as various modifications need to be made depending on the presenting clinical scenario. All the forms of the extended exenteration are various modifications of the total lid sparing orbital exenteration as described above. We discuss step by step approach in different clinical scenarios depending on the extension of the cancer into various surrounding structures.

7. Orbital exenteration with surrounding skin and soft tissue resection

The demonstrated patient has a pleomorphic rhabdomyosarcoma of the right orbit (**Figure 11**). Main bulk of the tumor was present in the superior orbit and protruded between the eyelids superiorly (**Figure 11**). The tumor was infiltrating the soft tissues of the eyelids circumferentially (**Figure 11**). He had received chemotherapy and radiation as part of initial treatment with disease progression. A preoperative contrast-enhanced CT scan axial and coronal view demonstrates well defined, homogenous and iso-dense soft tissue mass filling the orbit completely (**Figure 12**). The space occupying lesion was surrounding the globe completely with invasion of the subcutaneous soft tissues overlying the nasal bone and extends up to the lamina papyracea of the right orbit (**Figure 12A**). There was erosion of the floor of the orbit without extension of the disease into the maxilla (**Figure 12B**).

Assessment of the surrounding skin and soft tissue is done by palpation and lifting of the skin from the underlying structures before marking the incision. Radiology images are carefully reviewed, preferably with radiologist and incision planned accordingly. In this particular case, significant amount of eyelid tissue is infiltrated by the tumor and eyelid preservation is not possible, the incisions here

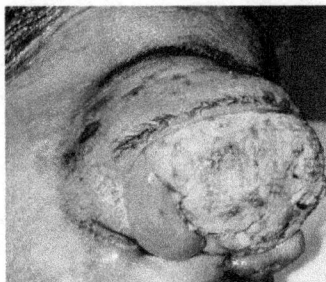

Figure 11.
Advanced pleomorphic rhabdomyosarcoma of the right orbit fungating through the palpebral fissure and invasion of the surrounding skin and soft tissues.

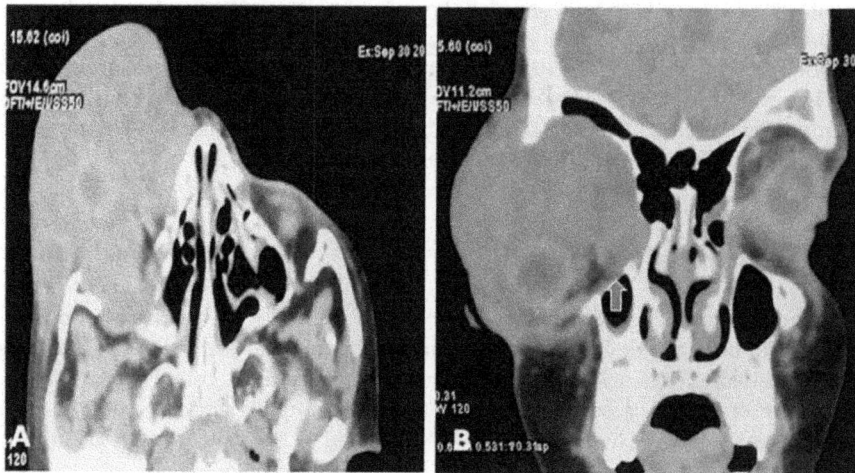

Figure 12.
(A) The axial view of contrast enhanced CT scan shows a large soft-tissue homogenous, iso-dense mass involving all the quadrants of the orbit enclosing the globe in middle with eyelid and surrounding soft tissue infiltration. (B) The coronal view of contrast enhanced CT scan shows a large soft-tissue homogenous, iso-dense mass involving all the quadrants of the orbit with eyelid and surrounding soft tissue infiltration.

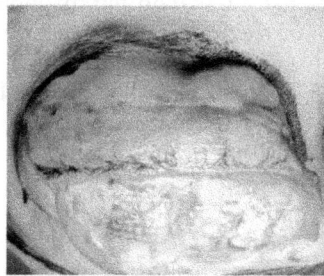

Figure 13.
Eyelid sacrificing skin incision marked for the planned surgical excision in case of involvement of the eyelids.

is made full thickness along the orbital rim area at least 1 cm away from the indurated skin margin (**Figure 13**). Incision is then made along the skin marking, full thickness, as demonstrated, in small increments and complete hemostasis achieved in incised segments to reduce the blood loss and maintain clean surgical field (**Figure 14A**). This procedure is continued circumferentially 360 degrees along the planned incision (**Figure 14B**). Once the orbital rim is reached, periosteum is exposed and a fine tip monopolar cutting cautery is used to incise the periosteum circumferentially just outside the orbital rim or arcus marginalis (**Figure 15A** and **B**). After incision of periosteum around the rim, Freer periosteal elevator is used to dissect the periosteum off the bony orbit circumferentially (**Figure 16A** and **B**). After elevation of the periosteum circumferentially, subperiosteal dissection continued till the orbital apex (**Figure 17A** and **B**). Rest of the steps are similar to the total lid sparing orbital exenteration as described above. The lacrimal sac is approached by dissecting medial to it and dividing common canaliculi and orbicularis attachments. It is then dissected from the lacrimal sac fossa and divided from the nasolacrimal duct, preferably with cautery (**Figure 18A** and **B**). The exposed nasolacrimal duct is obliterated by cautery to

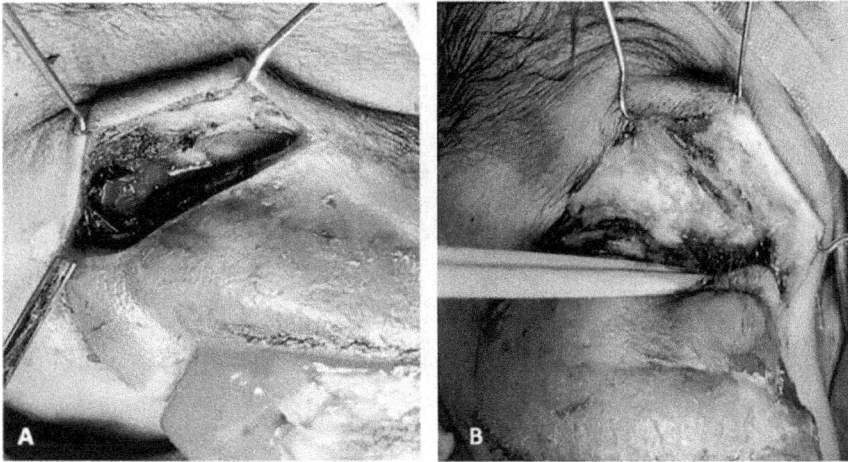

Figure 14.
(A) The skin incision is full thickness and is deepened in a plane superficial to the periosteum in small increments to achieve complete hemostasis. (B) Skin incision is deepened up to the periosteum circumferentially 360° around the orbit.

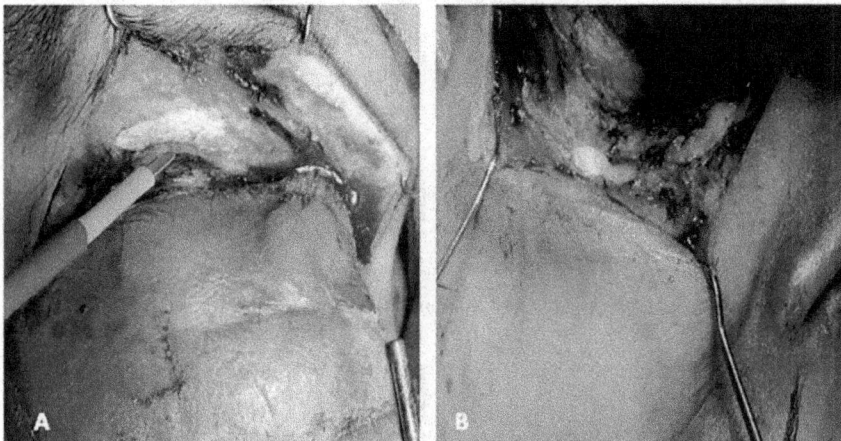

Figure 15.
(A) Periosteum is incised with monopolar cautery along the orbital rim superiorly. (B) Periosteum is incised with monopolar cautery just beyond the orbital rim inferiorly again 360° circumferentially.

decrease the risk of fistula formation. A pair of curved enucleation scissors are then introduced into the posterior orbit and the optic nerve, superior orbital fissure contents and posterior orbital tissues are cut (**Figure 19A**). The socket is carefully examined carefully for any residual tumor tissue (**Figure 19B**). In such a case where generous amount of the eyelids have been sacrificed due to the tumor infiltration, different local or free flaps may be used for reconstruction. Since our case was child of 11 years age, we preferred generous undermining of the surrounding skin flaps (**Figure 20A** and **B**) and could approximate primarily, albeit with some tension (**Figure 21**). Our preference is always to close the orbit with preserved lids or advancement of the cheek skin to decrease the donor site morbidity.

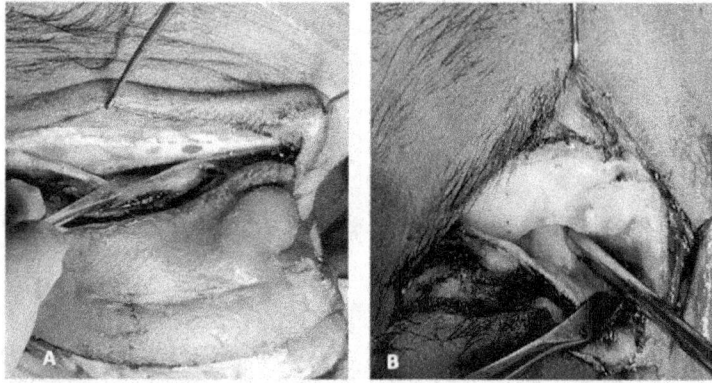

Figure 16.
(A and B) Freer periosteal elevator is used to elevate the periosteum of the orbit circumferentially.

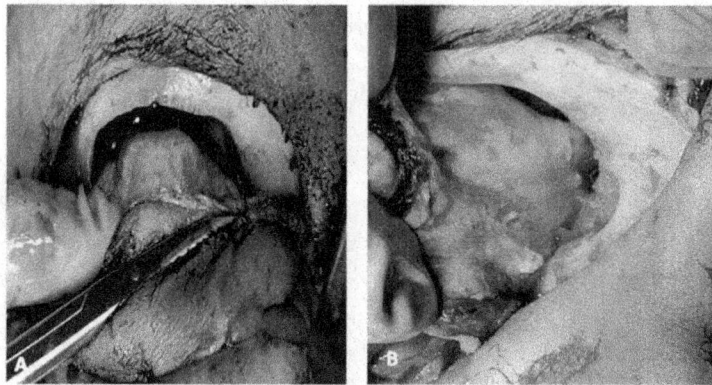

Figure 17.
(A and B) Subperiosteal dissection being carried to the orbital apex.

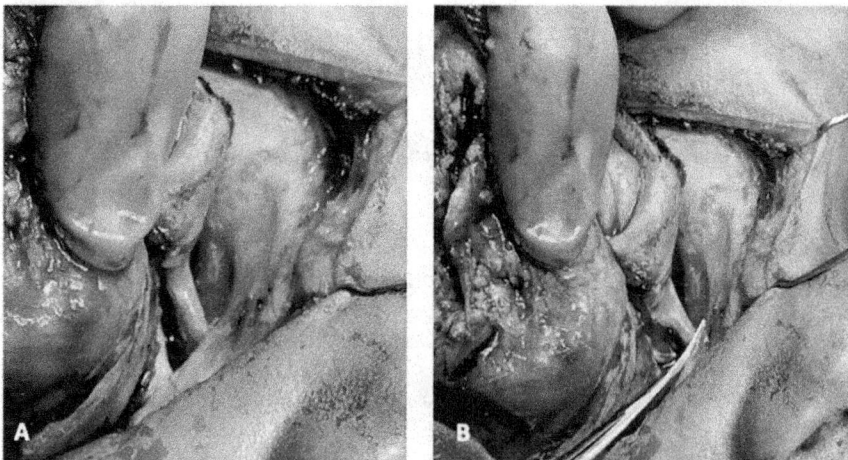

Figure 18.
(A) Lacrimal sac is approached by dissecting medial to it and dividing common canaliculi and orbicularis attachments. (B) Lacrimal sac dissected from the fossa and divided from the nasolacrimal duct.

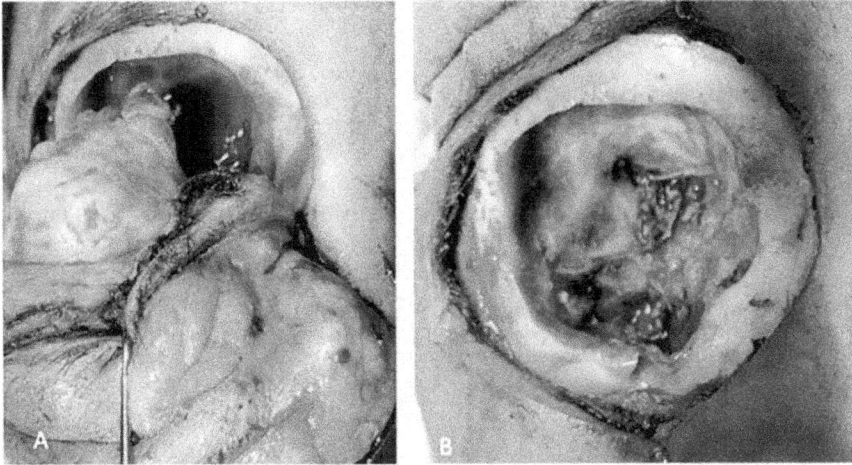

Figure 19.
(A) The extraocular muscles and the optic nerve are divided at the orbital apex with curved enucleation scissors and specimen delivered. (B) Empty socket after orbital exenteration.

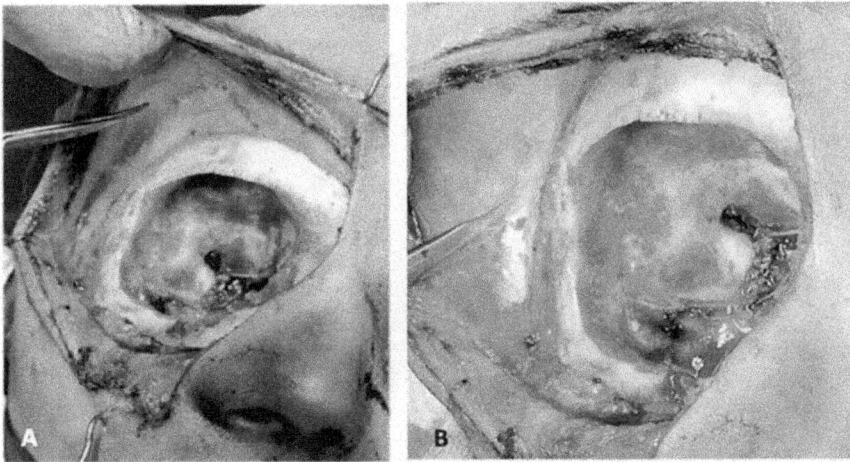

Figure 20.
(A) Generous undermining of the superior skin flap with pericranium kept undisturbed on cranium. (B) Generous undermining of the lateral skin flap.

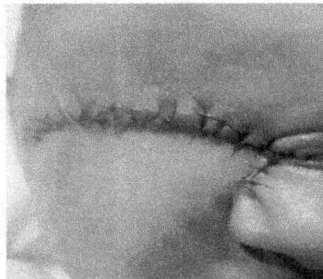

Figure 21.
Primary closure of the surgical defect.

8. Radical resection for a locally advanced basal cell carcinoma involving floor of the orbit and zygomatic bone

This demonstrated case has long standing basal cell carcinoma of the left lower eyelid with extension into the orbit (**Figure 22**). The CT scan showed soft tissue mass with enhancement involving left lateral eyelid skin and subcutaneous tissue with extension to the pre-septal and post-septal left orbit. The lesion invades anterior portion of the floor of the orbit and zygomatic bone (**Figure 23**). The plan of surgical resection includes access through upper eyelid preservation with upper eyelid incision marked 2 mm beyond the eyelash margin, while on the lower lid the involved skin and soft tissue is generously resected en-bloc with the specimen (**Figure 24**). The upper lid dissection is done between anterior and posterior lamella of the eyelid, while the lower lid incision is full thickness at least 1 cm away from the visible tumor margin. The skin incision is deepened, leaving a generous amount of soft tissue on the lateral and inferior wall of the orbit to secure adequate margins around the tumor. The skin flap is elevated laterally, directly over the zygoma and the anterior bony wall of the maxilla. The upper lid dissection and periosteal elevation is similar to the steps described for above first case. The bone cuts to encompass the tumor are depicted on a skull (**Figures 25** and **26**). A power saw is used to make bone cuts for the proposed inferior orbital wall and zygoma resection. The inferior

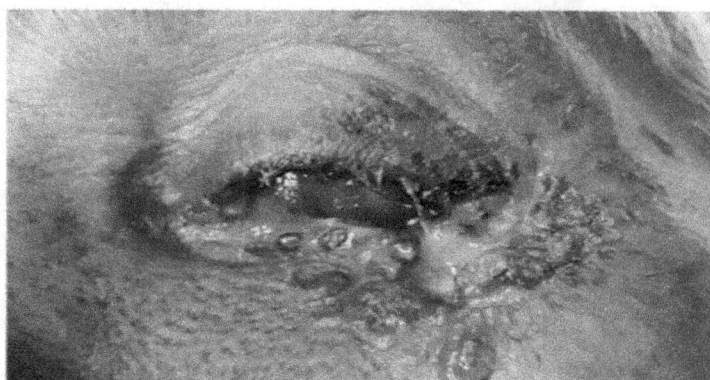

Figure 22.
Basal cell carcinoma of the left lateral lower eyelid with orbital invasion.

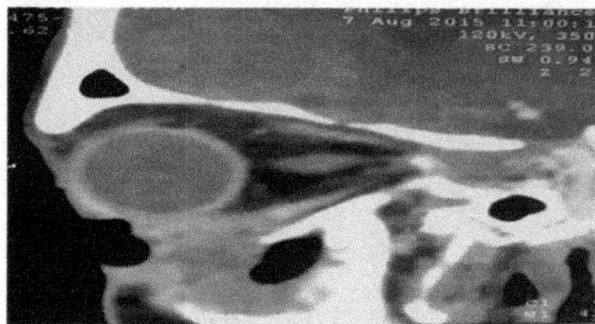

Figure 23.
CT scan showing orbital invasion by periocular basal cell carcinoma. Erosion of the orbital rim and floor is noticed.

rim of the orbit is divided medial to the infraorbital foramen to keep the lower lateral quadrant with the specimen with adequate bone margins (**Figure 25**). This bone cut extends through the floor of the orbit up to the optic foramen posteriorly. Bone cuts are made on the lateral wall of the orbit at fronto-zygomatic suture and zygomatico-temporal suture (**Figure 26**). This superior bone cut is extended through to the superior orbital fissure (**Figure 25**). Small osteotomes are used to

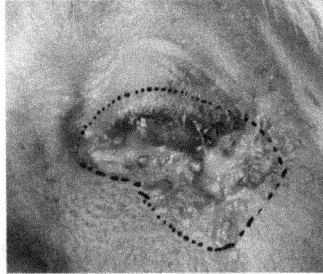

Figure 24.
The plan of surgical resection through a upper lid sparing, while generous amount of skin and soft tissues are kept on lower lateral region.

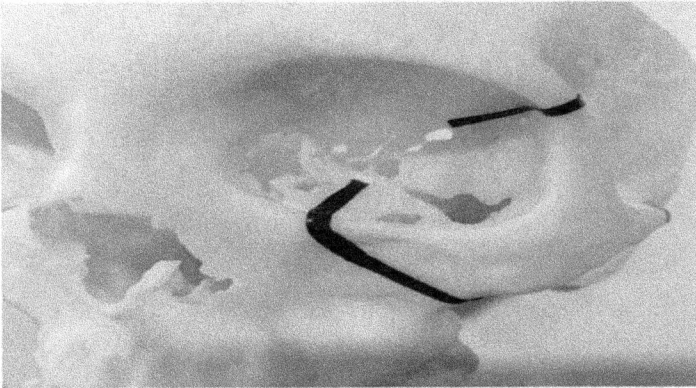

Figure 25.
The inferior rim of the orbit is divided medial to the infraorbital foramen.

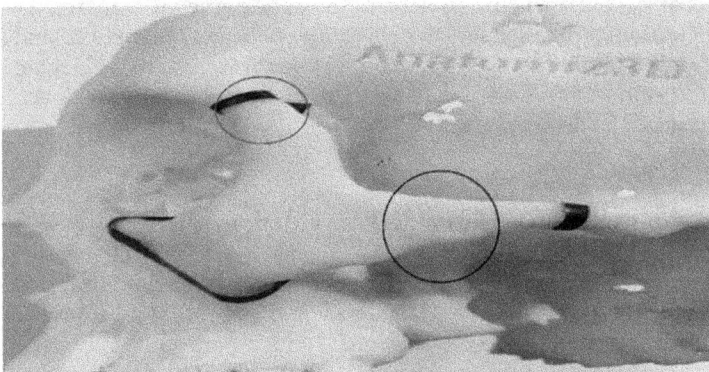

Figure 26.
Bone cuts are made on the lateral wall of the orbit at fronto-zygomatic suture (blue circle) and zygomatico-temporal suture (black circle).

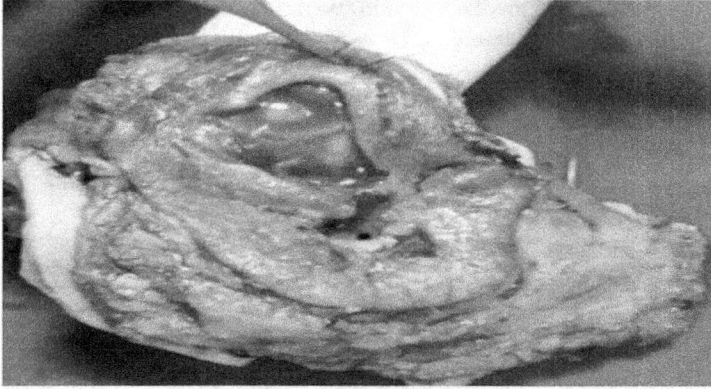

Figure 27.
Anterior view of the total orbital exenteration and lateral orbital wall resection specimen.

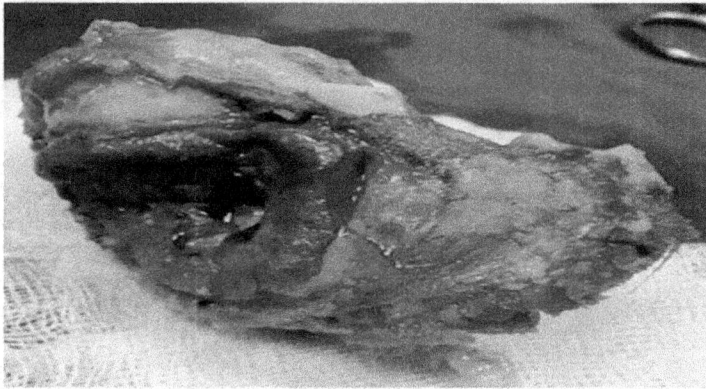

Figure 28.
Lateral view of the total orbital exenteration and lateral wall removal specimen.

complete the bone cuts and to mobilize the bony attachments of the surgical specimen. Once all bone cuts are completed, the surgical specimen remains attached only
at the cone of the orbit posteriorly through the attachments of the extraocular muscles and the optic nerve. The orbital contents are retracted laterally and the posterior
attachments of the extraocular muscles and the optic nerve are transacted with
curved enucleation curved scissors to deliver the specimen (**Figures 27** and **28**).
Rest of the steps are similar to as described for the above case for achieving
hemostasis. Specimen and orbital defect is examined after hemostasis is achieved and
reconstruction of the defect done.

9. Orbital exenteration with medial maxillectomy

Orbital exenteration with addition of the operative procedure to include part of
maxilla is used when the orbital tumors invade adjacent ethmoid sinuses or the
nasolacrimal duct system. Various additional surgical procedures are used to
remove such tumors depending on the clinical scenario. The demonstrated patient
shown in **Figure 29**, has lympho-epithelial carcinoma of the left lacrimal sac. An
axial T1-weighted magnetic resonance imaging (MRI) scan, reveals a multi-lobular,
slightly hyperintense lesion in the medial aspect of the right orbit with loss of plane

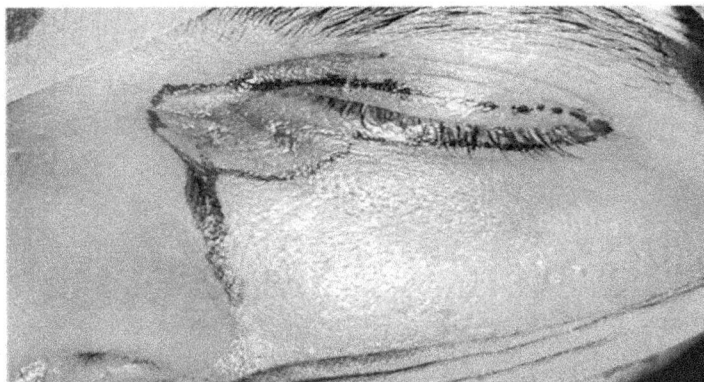

Figure 29.
Clinical picture of lymphoepithelial carcinoma of the left lacrimal sac. Incision encompasses the involved portion of the skin overlying the lacrimal fossa.

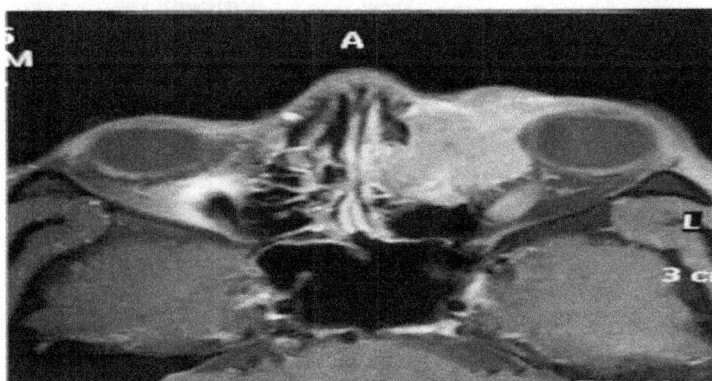

Figure 30.
An axial T1-weighted MRI scan, reveals a multi-lobular, slightly hyperintense lesion in the medial aspect of the right orbit with loss of plane with medial rectus.

with medial rectus (**Figure 30**). An axial T2-weighted MRI scan demonstrates space occupying mass in the medial orbit with extension to the ethmoid sinuses (**Figure 31**). An axial view post-contrast fat-suppressed T1-weighted image shows peripheral enhancement and a lack of central enhancement (**Figure 32**). The operative procedure therefore will entail an orbital exenteration with a medial maxillectomy. The medial wall of maxilla is accessed through lateral rhinotomy incision that extends from the floor of the nasal cavity along the alar groove and the lateral aspect of the nose up to the medial canthus. Upper and lower eyelid incisions are made 2 mm away from the lid margin and are extended along the nasolabial fold to encompass the involved portion of the skin overlying the lacrimal fossa and nasolacrimal duct (**Figure 29**). Skin incision and flap elevation up to the periosteum is done as described above in the first case except that a generous portion of soft tissue is sacrificed at the medial aspect of the incision where the skin is involved. Here the skin incision is deepened straight down to the nasal bone medially and the anterior wall of the maxilla laterally. In the inferomedial quadrant of the orbit the soft tissues along the lacrimal sac region are retained on the specimen. No attempt is made to mobilize the periosteum on the lower medial wall of the orbit at the lacrimal apparatus and the lacrimal fossa as medial wall of maxilla will be resected en-bloc with the orbital contents. At the lower end of pyriform aperture of the nose

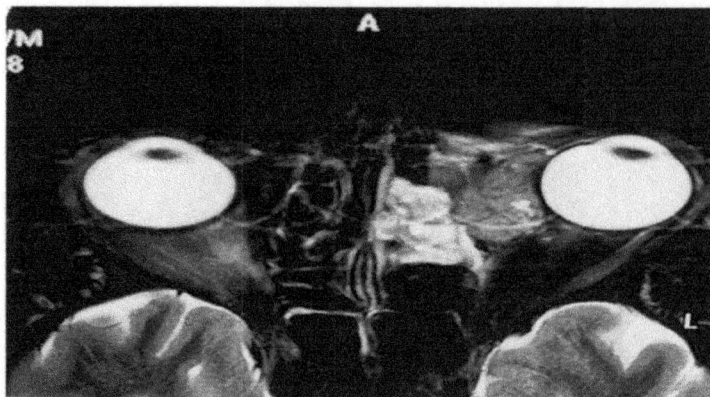

Figure 31.
An axial T2-weighted MRI scan demonstrates mass lesion in the medial orbit extending to the ethmoid sinuses.

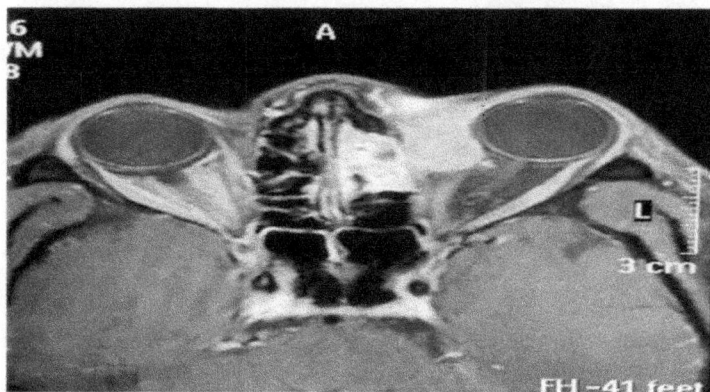

Figure 32.
An axial view postcontrast fat-suppressed T1-weighted image shows peripheral enhancement with lack of central enhancement.

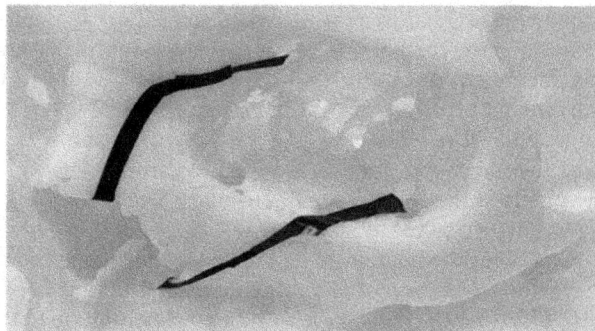

Figure 33.
The planned bone cuts are outlined on a skull superior cut is along the nasal bone and inferior cut is made lateral to the inferior orbital foramen.

mucosal incision is made with the monopolar cautery till the posterior choana below the inferior turbinate. After periosteal elevation of the superior, lateral and the inferior orbital walls, a oscillating power saw is used to make bone cuts for the proposed medial maxillectomy (**Figure 33**). The inferior rim of the orbit is divided

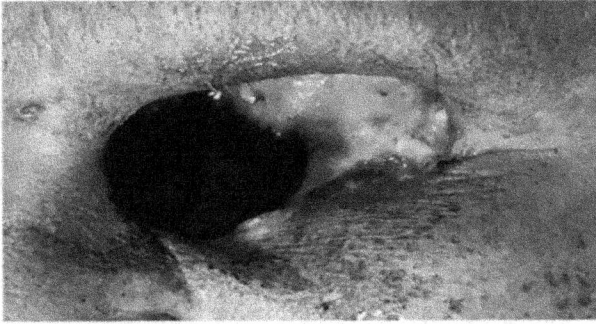

Figure 34.
The postoperative appearance of the patient approximately 2 month after surgery shows excellent healing within the orbital socket.

lateral to the infraorbital foramen to keep the lower medial quadrant in the specimen with adequate bone margins. This bone cut extends through the floor of the orbit up to the inferior orbital fissure and the anterior wall of the maxilla is divided in the plane extending up to the pyriform aperture (**Figure 33**). Superior bone cut is made above the meridian of the orbit so that entire lacrimal fossa can be resected with the specimen with satisfactory margins. This extends posteriorly along the lamina papyracea up to the posterior ethmoids. Medial bone cut is made on the lateral aspect of the left nasal bone from the orbit up to the nasal vestibule (**Figure 33**). Inferiorly along the pyriform aperture, osteotome is used to make a bone cut along the lower border of the lateral wall of the nose, below the inferior turbinate. Once all the osteotomies are completed, the surgical specimen remains attached only at the cone of the orbit posteriorly through the attachments of the extraocular muscles and the optic nerve. Rest of the steps are similar as described above. Additional attention is paid to the sphenopalatine artery as brisk hemorrhage may result from it and is easily controlled with electrocoagulation. In this particular case due to adjuvant radiotherapy, necrosis of the skin flaps resulted in the open orbital defect (**Figure 34**). The surgical defect following healing of the socket shows the medial one-third of the orbital rim has been resected to encompass the tumor of the lacrimal apparatus, which is removed in an en bloc fashion with the contents of the orbit and lateral wall of the nasal cavity (**Figure 34**). Such cases can be rehabilitated best by prosthetic replacement and glasses as shown in the **Figure 35** and **Figure 48**.

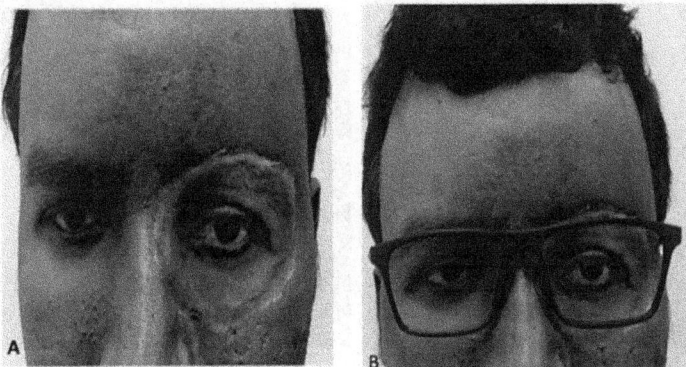

Figure 35.
(A) Rehabilitation of the orbital socket with prosthesis. (B) Glasses are used to enhance appearance.

10. Orbital exenteration with lateral wall removal

This patient has right lateral canthal infiltrative basal cell carcinoma with lateral orbital wall invasion (**Figure 36**). He had been operated twice before and had also received radiotherapy as part of initial treatment. Coronal view CT scan revealed ill-defined soft tissue mass causing erosion of the lateral wall and infiltration of the orbit and globe (**Figure 37A** and **B**). The surgical plan is orbital exenteration with lateral wall removal along with surrounding soft tissues. Upper and lower lid incisions were marked 2 mm beyond eyelid margin with generous amount of skin and soft tissue kept attached to the eyelids at the lateral canthus to ensure satisfactory soft tissue margins (**Figure 38**). Superior lid, inferior lid and medial dissection is done similarly as described in first case, while laterally generous amount of soft tissues is left for safe margin attached to the specimen. Superiorly, medially and inferiorly subperiosteal dissection is done till the orbital apex as described for above cases. The surgical procedure needs a orbito-zygomatic cranial base exposure. A superior, lateral and inferior orbitectomy is done along with the removal of the zygomatic bone as shown on the skull (**Figure 39A** and **B**). Oscillating saw is used to make bone cuts from the superior orbital rim to superior orbital fissure posteriorly. Inferior cut is made from the inferior orbital rim to the inferior orbital fissure

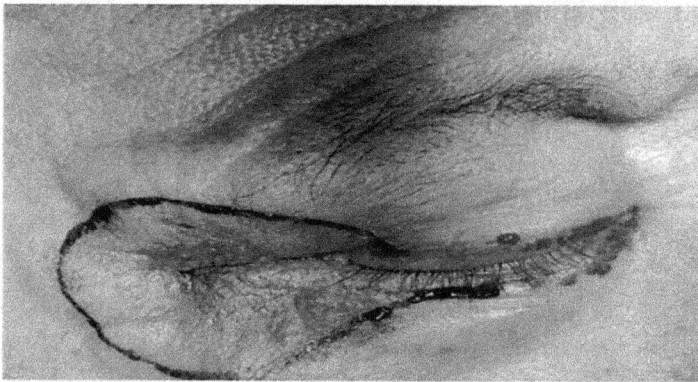

Figure 36.
A patient with a basal cell carcinoma of the right lateral canthus with extension into the orbit.

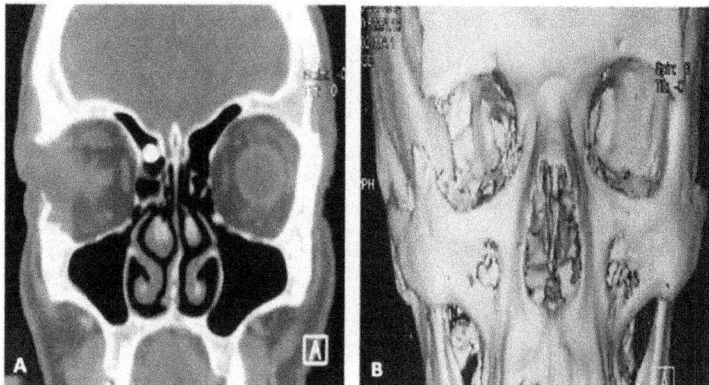

Figure 37.
(A) The coronal view of the CT scan shows ill-defined tumor involving the lateral quadrant of the right orbit with erosion of the lateral wall. (B) 3-D reconstruction of the orbit showing eroded lateral wall.

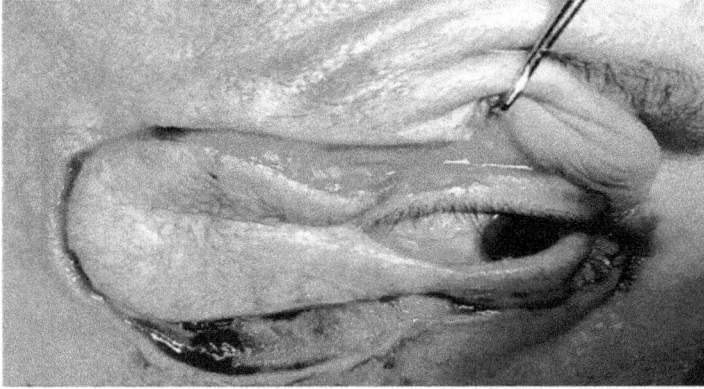

Figure 38.
Surgical plan of resection with generous amount of soft tissues kept on the lateral wall to achieve disease free margins.

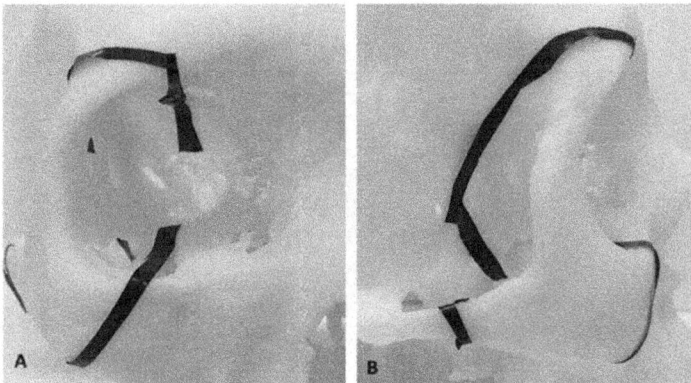

Figure 39.
(A) Anterior view of the planned bone cuts outlined on a skull. (B) Right lateral view of the planned bone cuts outlined on a skull.

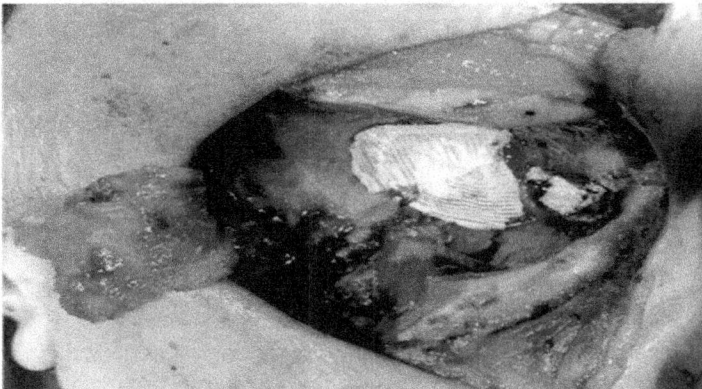

Figure 40.
The surgical defect shows the apex of the orbit and remnant walls after resection.

posteriorly and zygomatico - temporal suture is divided. Small osteotomes are used to mobilize the surgical specimen after division of the surrounding soft tissues with electro- cautery. Diamond bur can be used to smoothen the bone edges. In a

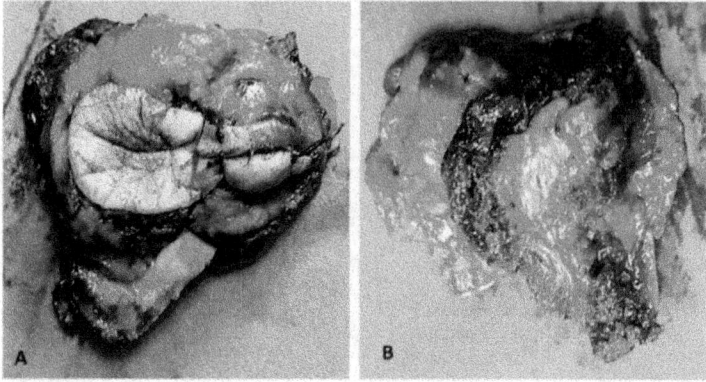

Figure 41.
(A) Anterior view of the surgical specimen shows en-bloc resection of the tumor with the contents of the orbit and the lateral soft tissues. (B) Posterior view of the surgical specimen shows en-bloc resection of the tumor with the contents of the orbit and the lateral soft tissues.

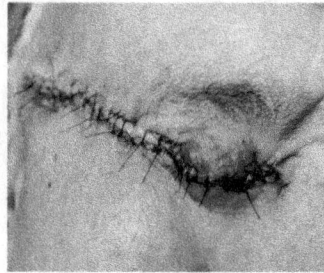

Figure 42.
The skin incision is closed in layers.

scenario of the erosion of the cranial base in the region, diamond bur can be used to remove the bone without causing tear in the dura. Even appropriate size Kerrison's punch can be used to remove the cranial base with adequate margins with out injuring dura. The surgical defect after removal of the specimen is examined for completion of surgery (**Figure 40**) and specimen can be sent for frozen section analysis of soft tissue margins. Anterior and posterior view of the specimen can be seen in the **Figure 41A** and **B**. In this particular case since enough of upper and lower eyelid flaps could be preserved, we could achieve primary closure (**Figure 42**).

11. Orbital exenteration with superior orbital margin/frontal bone removal

The patient presented with adenoid cystic carcinoma of the right lacrimal gland (**Figure 43**). Contrast enhanced CT scan coronal and axial view reveals soft tissue mass in the upper lateral and superior orbit with outward and medial displacement of the eye ball (**Figure 44A** and **B**). Three dimensional reconstruction reveals erosion of the superior orbital rim and outer plate of the frontal bone without any intracranial extension (**Figure 45**). Such a case in addition to the orbital exenteration will need lateral and superior orbitectomy. Skin incision and periosteum exposure were performed as described for the first case. The periosteum on the superior rim was removed widely to encompass the involved area and achieve negative margins of resection. After orbital exenteration the lateral and the superior orbital

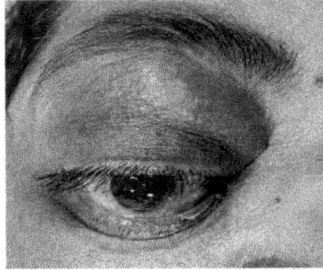

Figure 43.
This patient has an adenoid-cystic carcinoma of the right lacrimal gland.

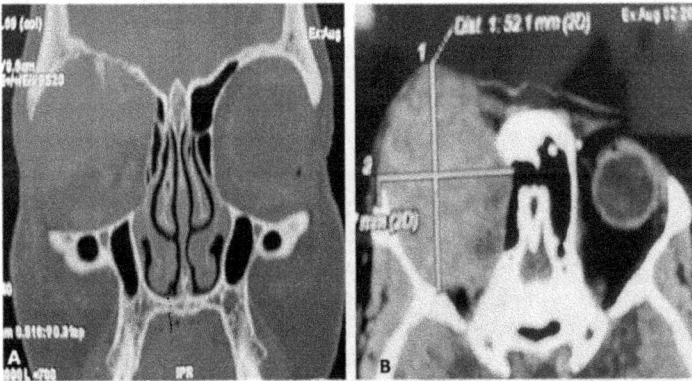

Figure 44.
(A) A contrast-enhanced coronal view of CT scan shows the tumor involving the superior and lateral orbit with displacement of the globe. (B) A contrast-enhanced axial view of CT scan shows the tumor involving the orbit.

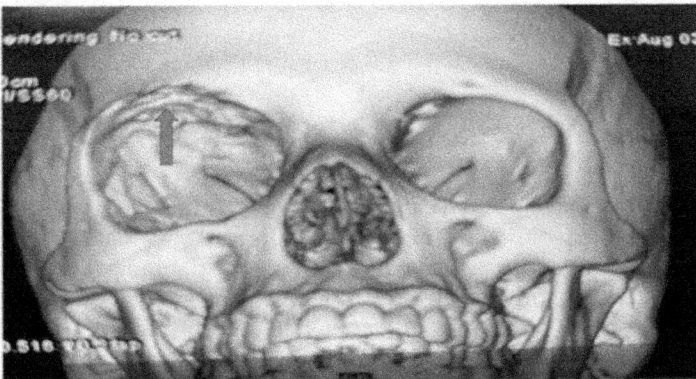

Figure 45.
3-D reconstruction revealed erosion of the orbital rim and outer plate of the frontal bone.

wall or cranial base was drilled generously to expose dura completely to ensure even the microscopic tumor is removed. The skull base area to be resected is shown in the **Figure 46A** and **B**. The Bone drilling is done well beyond the grossly involved margin and dura exposed (**Figure 47**). To hasten the process Kerrison's punch can be used to remove the thinned out bone. Since this is an eyelid sparing procedure, surgical defect is repaired with closure of the remnant eyelid flaps.

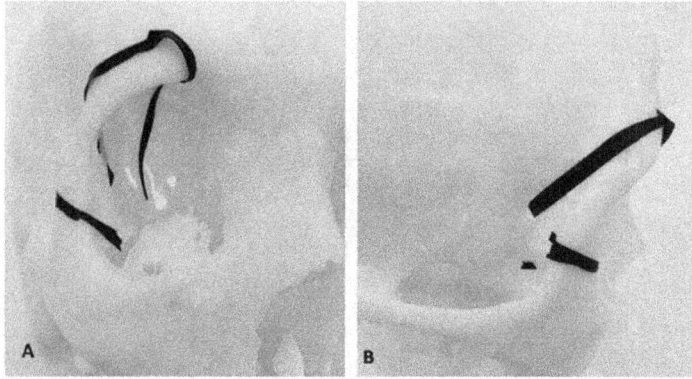

Figure 46.
(A) Anterior view of the planned bone cuts outlined on a skull. (B) Right lateral view of the planned bone cuts outlined on a skull.

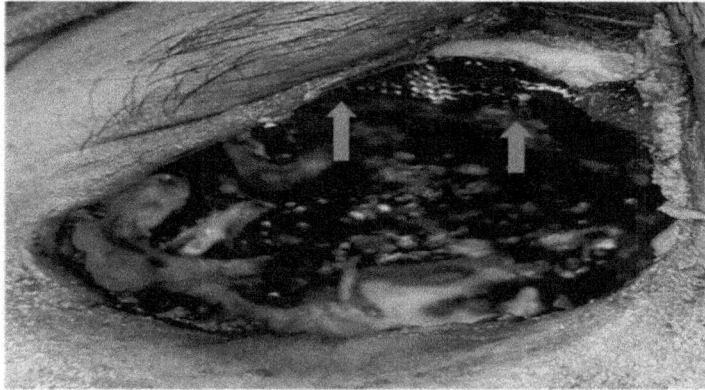

Figure 47.
The surgical defect shows the complete removal of the superior and lateral wall of the orbit and exposed dura (arrow).

12. Orbital exenteration with total maxillectomy

This patient has squamous cell carcinoma of the right maxillary sinus invading the orbit through the periosteum (**Figure 48**). Contrast enhanced CT scan of the paranasal sinuses reveals soft tissue mass involving the right maxillary sinus completely and eroding floor of the orbit and extending into the orbit through the periosteum (**Figure 49**). To remove the tumor en-bloc, orbital exenteration with total maxillectomy is indicated. Orbital exenteration of a functioning eye with normal vision is only indicated if the procedure is done with curative intention. A lateral rhinotomy incision with midline lip is split is extended laterally as upper and lower lid incisions circumferentially encompassing the palpebral fissure of the eye (**Figure 48**). The skin incision begins in the midline of the upper lip up to the root of the columella. Here the incision extends into the floor of the nasal cavity and then returns back outside of the nasal cavity around the ala of the nose up to the medial canthus to join circumferential orbital incision (**Figure 48**). The skin incision is deepened through the subcutaneous tissues and musculature of the upper lip and the right cheek. The cheek flap is elevated laterally with a mucosal incision along the upper gingivobuccal sulcus. The skin incision for the sub-ciliary extension begins at

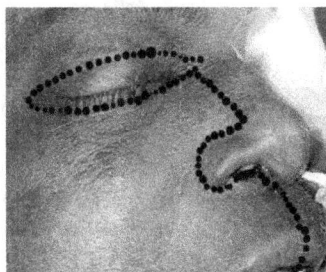

Figure 48.
Clinical picture of advanced squamous cell carcinoma of the right maxillary sinus invading right orbit.

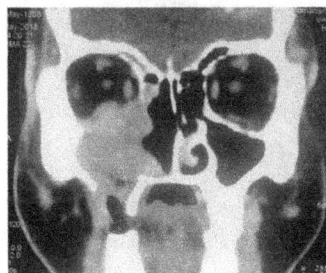

Figure 49.
Coronal CT scans show a large left maxillary sinus mass that has destroyed most of the sinus walls. The tumor extends into the orbit through the periosteum.

about the level of the medial canthus of the eye 2 mm beyond the eyelid margin. The skin incision here should be placed meticulously without tearing as the skin over the eyelid is thin. The cheek flap is elevated to about 1 cm beyond the lateral canthus to provide adequate access to the anterolateral wall of the maxilla. After elevation of the cheek flap, attachment of the orbital periosteum to the orbital rim is incised in its superior half. A periosteal elevator is used to separate the orbital periosteum from the bony roof of the orbit all the way up to the apex of the orbit. Periosteum of the lower half of the orbit is kept intact, so as not to violate the surgical field. The attachment of the masseter muscle on the inferior border of the zygoma is divided next with use of the cautery.

A mouth gag is placed on the contralateral side to open the oral cavity and a tongue depressor is used to depress the tongue. A mucosal incision is made between the lateral incisor and the canine tooth, which marks the anterior line of resection of the alveolar process of the maxilla. An incision is now made in the mucosa of the hard palate along midline from the junction of the soft and hard palate and it is further extended to the incision of the alveolar process between the canine and lateral incisor (**Figure 51**). Posterior end of the midline palatal incision is turned laterally behind the maxillary tubercle to connect the upper gingivobuccal-sulcus incision. This incision is deepened through the mucoperiosteum of the hard palate. Posteriorly the incision is deepened through the attachments of the medial ptery-goid muscle to free up soft-tissue attachments to the maxilla.

Nasal vestibule is opened through the piriform aperture to expose the nasal process of the maxilla. All the soft tissue attachment of the maxilla and the orbit are thoroughly divided before proceeding for bone cuts. All the bone cuts are marked by electrocautery. Superior bone cut is through the nasal process of maxilla, later-ally the maxilla is separated from the zygomatic arch along the inferior orbital fissure and inferiorly the maxilla is divided through its alveolar process between the lateral incisor and canine tooth up to the midline to the posterior margin and from there onward through the midline up to its posterior margin (**Figures 50** and **51**). Posterolateral wall is separated from the pterygoid plates through its hamulus by placing a curved osteotome in between and gentle tap with mallet (**Figure 52**). All the bone cuts are accomplished by oscillating power saw. Once all the bone cuts are completed with the power saw, an osteotome is used to mobilize the specimen en-bloc (**Figures 53–55**). Soft-tissue and muscular attachments on the posterior aspect of the maxilla are divided with heavy curved scissors. The surgical defect

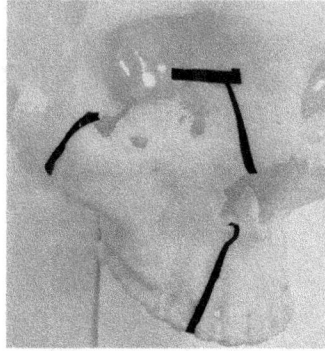

Figure 50.
Medial and lateral bone cuts shown on skull.

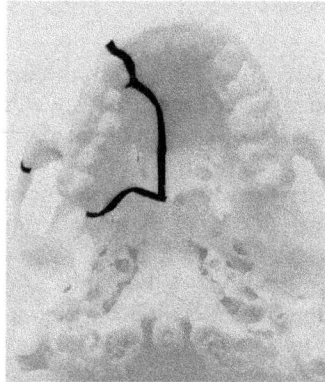

Figure 51.
Palatal bone cuts shown on skull.

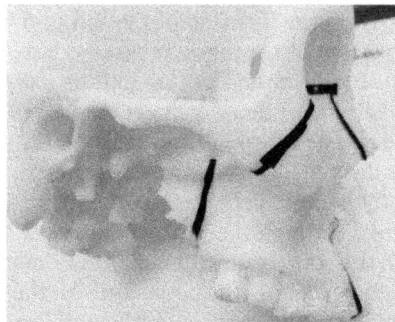

Figure 52.
Posterior separation line between maxilla and pterygoid plates.

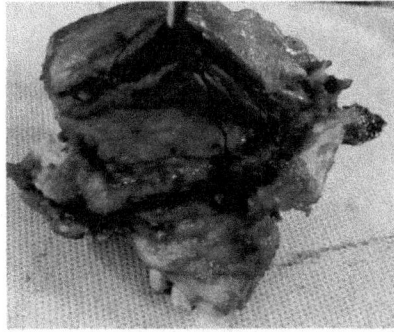

Figure 53.
A anterolateral view of the specimen.

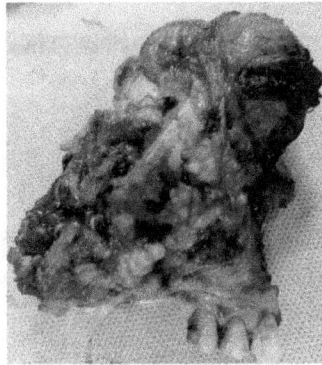

Figure 54.
A lateral view of the specimen.

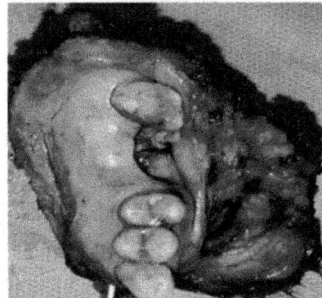

Figure 55.
A palatal view of the specimen.

following total maxillectomy with orbital exenteration is shown is shown in (**Figures 55** and **56**). Surgical defect was reconstructed by primary closure and prosthetic rehabilitation (**Figure 57**).

13. Reconstruction following extended orbital exenteration

Reconstruction of the defects that result from extended orbital exenteration is a challenge. There are basically two methods, first is open method and second is closed method (**Table 4**). In open method, healing occurs by secondary

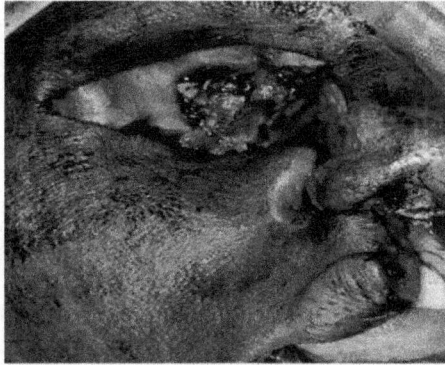

Figure 56.
Surgical defect with cheek flap.

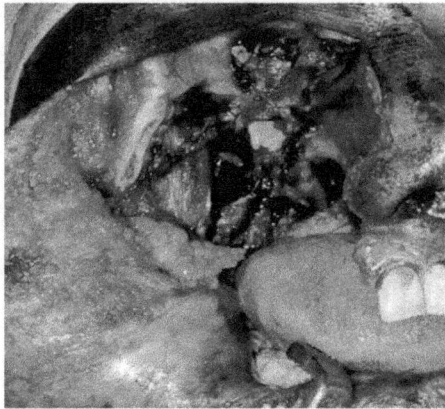

Figure 57.
Surgical defect with retracted cheek flap.

Technique	
Open method	Healing by secondary intension
	Split thickness skin graft
	Dermis-fat graft
Closed method	Locoregional flaps
	Residual preserved lids Cheek advancement flaps Regional pedicle flaps Temporalis muscle transfer Frontalis rotational flap Temporoparietal fascial flap
	Distant flaps
	Microvascular: Radial forearm falp Anterolateral thigh flap Rectus abdominis flap

Table 4.
Reconstruction of the orbital cavity.

intention, as the depth of the orbit is left open for granulation with regular dressings [18]. This is time consuming process and this option is suboptimal if the patient is to have postoperative radiation which in most cases needs to be started within 4 weeks post-surgery [18]. Other option is to layer the orbital cavity with a split thickness skin graft. It is usually harvested from the thigh with a humby's knife or a dermatome, placed directly on the bone and sutured to the skin edges around the socket. It maintains a deeper socket in comparison to the secondary healing as it reduces wound contracture. Due to donor site morbidity and failure of graft uptake in particularly diabetic patients, split thickness grafts are used in conjunction with other flaps like pericranial periosteal flaps from forehead. Since pericranial are vascular, it enhances the uptake of split thickness skin graft.

In Closed method of reconstruction, the orbital cavity is reconstructed either with the residual preserved lid, cheek advancement, locoregional flaps or microvascular free tissue transfer [19–30]. We prefer to close orbit directly in case of adequate amount of lid tissue has been preserved or with cheek advancement. It is the modification of the cervicofacial flap and offers a one-stage, reliable, and safe method of reconstruction following orbital exenteration [19]. Subcutaneous cheek dissection can be performed to various levels usually to a level just below the oral commissure and 2–3 cm below the angle of the mandible avoiding injury to the branches of facial nerve. It can also be used in conjunction with other methods of reconstruction like peri-cranial flap. Other loco-regional options include: a cheek fascio-cutaneous V-Y flap, galeal flap, pericranial flap, cutaneous flap from the forehead and temporalis muscle flap [31–33]. Cutaneous forehead flap based on the frontal branch of the temporal artery described by Rodrigues ML et al. can be used effective to cover the orbital defect [20]. Apart from being a single stage procedure, this flap can obliterate the orbital defect immediately and adequately [20]. This method is easy, less time consuming and flap has a reliable blood supply and is reproducible. In cases where lateral orbital wall has also been resected, temporalis muscle flap can be used to reconstruct the orbital defect [21]. Menon NG et al. illustrated the method where temporalis muscle can be used to reconstruct the orbital defect with intact lateral wall of the orbit [30]. They transposed entire temporalis muscle to orbit after creating a large window in the lateral orbit, without resection of the lateral orbital rim [30]. Prefabricated myocutaneous - temporalis muscle flap was describe by Altindas M et al. for the reconstruction of eyelids and periorbital skin [22]. Scalp skin island is kept attached to the temporalis muscle for the reconstruction of lid margins and eyelashes and the neighboring bare temporoparietal fascia is used for the augmentation of the periorbital soft tissues [22]. Microvascular free tissue transfer is the ideal reconstructive option for the large and complex defects particularly resulting from extended orbital exenterations. Various free flaps like anterolateral thigh, radial fore-arm, parascapular, rectus abdominis muscle and gracilis muscle free flaps have been described for orbital reconstruction [25–29]. The modified radial forearm flap described by Purnell et al. provides abundant thin, pliable tissue, facilitating resurfacing of the entire orbit [29].

All the reconstructive methods described till now provide a good cover only and prosthetic reconstruction is needed to improve the appearance beyond that of an eyepatch. Using only prothesis without osseointegration have drawback like poor fit and discoloration over time [33, 34]. With introduction of the osseo-integrated implants, there has been a significant improvement in fixation of prosthetics, with associated improvements in quality of life and compliance [35–40].

14. Conclusions

Extended orbital exenteration although highly disfiguring procedure give excellent chance of controlling the aggressive malignant process. A single procedure does not fit all the clinical scenarios. We have to examine the tumor extension and plan the procedure accordingly. There are many other clinical presentations like intracranial extension etc. We have purposefully restricted our discussion to only cases where dura was not infiltrated, for the readers to concentrate on the scenarios described above. Our efforts will continue to publish more such research to benefit our readers in understanding the surgical management of orbital tumors. Reconstruction of complex defects following extended orbital exenteration remain a challenge. Locoregional cutaneous and muscle flaps are useful, but free flaps like radial forearm flaps not only prove a good reconstruction option but tolerate the adjuvant treatment like radiation well. Last but not least, prosthesis helps in further enhancing the appearance and rehabilitation.

Acknowledgements

We are thankful to all the patients who have put trust in our abilities to treat them at our Apollo cancer center, Hyderabad, India. We are also grateful to Dr. Vijay Anand Reddy, Director Apollo cancer center, for constant encouragement to our scientific endeavors. This chapter would not have been possible without his valuable scientific inputs.

Conflict of interest

The authors declare no conflict of interest.

Author details

Arsheed Hussain Hakeem[1*], Hassaan Javaid[2], Novfa Iftikhar[3] and Usaamah Javaid[4]

1 Apollo Cancer Hospitals, Hyderabad, India

2 Department of Trauma Surgery, All India Institute of Medical Sciences, New Delhi, India

3 Department of Internal Medicine, Government Medical College, Srinagar, India

4 Department of Internal Medicine, Shadan Institute of Medical Sciences, Hyderabad, Telangana State, India

*Address all correspondence to: drahhakim@gmail.com

IntechOpen

References

[1] Payne JW, Duke JR, Butner R, Eifrig DE. Basal cell carcinoma of the eyelids. A long-term follow up study. Archives of Ophthalmology. 1969;**81**: 553-558

[2] Perlman GS, Hornblass A. Basal cell carcinoma of the eyelids: A review of patients treated by surgical excision. Ophthal Surg. 1976;**7**:23-27

[3] Howard GR, Nerad JA, Carter KD, Whitaker DC. Clinical characteristics associated with orbital invasion of cutaneous basal cell and squamous cell tumours of the eyelid. American Journal of Ophthalmology. 1992;**113**: 123-133

[4] Leibovitch I, McNab A, Sullivan T, Davis G, Selva D. Orbital invasion by periocular basal cell carcinoma. Ophthalmology. 2005;**112**:717-723

[5] Walling HW, Fosko SW, Geraminejad PA, Whitaker DC, Arpey CJ. Aggressive basal cell carcinoma: presentation, pathogenesis and management. Cancer Metastasis Reviews. 2004;**23**:389-402

[6] Savage RC. Orbital exenteration and reconstruction for massive basal cell and squamous cell carcinoma of cutaneous origin. Annals of Plastic Surgery. 1983; **10**(6):458-466

[7] Frezzoti R, Bonanni R, Nuti A, Polito E. Radical orbital resections. Advances in Ophthalmic Plastic and Reconstrctive Surgery. 1992;**9**:175-192

[8] Tyers AG. Orbital exenteration for invasive skin tumours. Eye (London, England). 2006;**20**:1165-1170

[9] Ben Simon GJ et al. Orbital exenteration: one size does not fit all. American Journal of Ophthalmology. 2005;**139**:11-17

[10] Goldberg RA, Kim JW, Shorr N. Orbital exenteration: Results of an individualized approach. Ophthalmic Plastic and Reconstructive Surgery. 2003;**19**:229-236

[11] Shields JA et al. Experience with eyelid-sparing orbital exenteration: The 2000 Tullos O. Coston Lecture. Ophthal Plast Reconstr Surg. 2001;**17**:355-361

[12] Gunalp I, Gunduz K, Duruk K. Orbital exenteration: A review of 429 cases. International Ophthalmology. 1995–1996;**19**(3):177-184

[13] Rathbun J, Beard C, Quickert MH. Evaluation of 48 cases of orbital exenteration. American Journal of Ophthalmology. 1971;**30**:191-199

[14] Bartley GB, Garrity JA, Waller RR, et al. Orbital exenteration at the Mayo Clinic 1967–1986. Ophthalmology. 1989; **96**(8):468–473

[15] Cook BE Jr, Bartley GB. Treatment options and future prospects for the management of eyelid malignancies: An evidence-based update. Ophthalmology. 2001;**108**:2088-2098

[16] McKelvie PA, Daniell M, McNab A, et al. Squamous cell carcinoma of the conjunctiva: A series of 26 cases. The British Journal of Ophthalmology. 2002; **86**:168-173

[17] Coston TO, Small RG. Orbital exenteration simplified. Transactions of the American Ophthalmological Society. 1981;**79**:136-152

[18] Putterman AM. Orbital exenteration with spontaneous granulation. Archives of Ophthalmology. 1986;**104**:139-140

[19] Sira M, Malhotra R. Reconstruction of orbital exenteration defects by primary closure using cheek

advancement. The British Journal of Ophthalmology. 2013;**97**:201-205

[20] Rodrigues ML, Kohler HF, Faria JC, et al. Reconstruction after extended orbital exenteration using a fronto-lateral flap. International Journal of Oral and Maxillofacial Surgery. 2009;**38**: 850-854

[21] Shipkov CD, Anastassov YC. Orbital reconstruction after exenteration with the whole transorbital temporalis muscle flap. Annals of Plastic Surgery. 2003;**51**:527

[22] Altindas M, Yucel A, Ozturk G, et al. The prefabricated temporal island flap for eyelid and eye socket reconstruction in total orbital exenteration patients: A new method. Annals of Plastic Surgery. 2010;**65**(9):177–182

[23] Lai A, Cheney ML. Temporoparietal fascial flap in orbital reconstruction. Archives of Facial Plastic Surgery. 2000; 2:196-201

[24] Rose EH, Norris MS. The versatile temporoparietal fascial flap: Adaptability to a variety of composite defects. Plastic and Reconstructive Surgery. 1990;**85**:224-232

[25] Li D, Jie Y, Liu H, et al. Reconstruction of anophthalmic orbits and contracted eye sockets with microvascular radial forearm free flaps. Ophthalmic Plastic and Reconstructive Surgery. 2008;**24**:94-97

[26] Lopez F, Suarez C, Carnero S, et al. Free flaps in orbital exenteration: A safe and effective method for reconstruction. European Archives of Oto-Rhino-Laryngology. 2013;**270**: 1947-1952

[27] Nicoli F, Chilgar RM, Sapountzis S, et al. Reconstruction after orbital exenteration using gracilis muscle free flap. Microsurgery. 2015;**35**(14): 169–176

[28] Pryor SG, Moore EJ, Kasperbauer JL. Orbital exenteration reconstruction with rectus abdominis microvascular free flap. Laryngoscope. 2005;**115**:1912-1916

[29] Purnell CA, Vaca EE, Ellis MF. Conical modification of forearm free flaps for single-stage reconstruction after Total orbital Exenteration. The Journal of Craniofacial Surgery. 2017; **28**(8):e767-e769

[30] Menon NG, Girotto JA, Goldberg NH, Silverman RP. Orbital Reconstruction After Exenteration: Use of a Transorbital Temporal Muscle Flap. Annals of Plastic Surgery. 2003;**50**(1): 38-42

[31] Moretti E, Ortiz S, Gómez García F, et al. Complete mobilization of the cheek zone for orbit exenteration. The Journal of Craniofacial Surgery. 2005; **16**:823-828

[32] Zwahlen RA, Gra¨tz KW, Obwegeser JA. The galea fascia flap in orbital reconstruction: Innovative harvest technique. European Journal of Surgical Oncology. 2006;**32**:804-807

[33] Cameron M, Gilbert PM, Mulhern MG, et al. Synchronous reconstruction of the exenterated orbit with a pericranial flap, skin graft and osseointegrated implants. Orbit. 2005; **24**:153-158

[34] Hanasono MM, Lee JC, Yang JS, et al. An algorithmic approach to reconstructive surgery and prosthetic rehabilitation after orbital exenteration. Plastic and Reconstructive Surgery. 2009;**123**:98-105

[35] Karakoca S, Aydin C, Yilmaz H, et al. Retrospective study of treatment outcomes with implant-retained extraoral prostheses: Survival rates and prosthetic complications. The Journal of Prosthetic Dentistry. 2010;**103**:118-126

[36] Arcuri MR, LaVelle WE, Fyler A, et al. Effects of implant anchorage on midface prostheses. The Journal of Prosthetic Dentistry. 1997;**78**:496-500

[37] Chang TL, Garrett N, Roumanas E, et al. Treatment satisfaction with facial prostheses. The Journal of Prosthetic Dentistry. 2005;**94**(22):275–280

[38] Karakoca Nemli S, Aydin C, Yilmaz H, et al. Retrospective study of implant-retained orbital prostheses: Implant survival and patient satisfaction. The Journal of Craniofacial Surgery. 2010;**21**(23):1178–1183

[39] Smolarz-Wojnowska A, Raithel F, Gellrich NC, et al. Quality of implant anchored craniofacial and intraoral prostheses: patient's evaluation. The Journal of Craniofacial Surgery. 2014; **25**(24):e202–e207

[40] Nemli SK, Aydin C, Yilmaz H, et al. Quality of life of patients with implant-retained maxillofacial prostheses: A prospective and retrospective study. The Journal of Prosthetic Dentistry. 2013;**109**:44-52

www.ingramcontent.com/pod-product-compliance
Lightning Source LLC
Chambersburg PA
CBHW081557190326
41458CB00015B/5635